Total Health
TALKING ABOUT LIFE'S CHANGES

Test and Quiz Master Book

Susan Boe

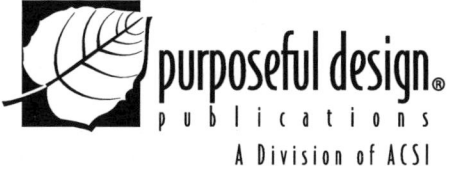

purposeful design®
PUBLICATIONS
A Division of ACSI

Colorado Springs, Colorado

Purposeful Design Publications is the publishing division of the Association of Christian Schools International (ACSI) and is committed to the ministry of Christian school education, to enable Christian educators and schools worldwide to effectively prepare students for life. As the publisher of textbooks, trade books, and other educational resources within ACSI, Purposeful Design Publications strives to produce biblically sound materials that reflect Christian scholarship and stewardship and that address the identified needs of Christian schools around the world.

Printed in the United States of America
16 15 14 13 12 11 10 09   5 6 7 8 9 10

Boe, Susan
    Total health: Talking about life's changes
    Second edition
    Total Health series
    ISBN 978-1-58331-234-6   Test and quiz master book   Catalog #7602

Cover design: Sarah E. Schultz

Purposeful Design Publications
A Division of ACSI
PO Box 65130 • Colorado Springs, CO 80962-5130
Customer Service: 800-367-0798 • www.acsi.org

Table of Contents

Test & Quiz Master Book

Total Health · Chapter 1 • Quiz A

Unit 1: Physical Health

Section 1.1

15 Points

Name:_____

Date: _____

Score: _____

MATCHING (5 points; 1 point each): For each numbered item, place the letter of the correct answer in the space provided at the left of each item. Each answer can be used only once.

1. _____ Habits
2. _____ Temptation
3. _____ Influences
4. _____ Deception
5. _____ Consequences

A. Something that allures or draws you especially to evil.
B. The outcome or result of something.
C. Music, the media, church, friends, and your relationship with God.
D. Patterns of how you will handle life's challenges.
E. To trick or mislead someone.

SHORT ANSWER: (10 points; 2 points each) Answer the following questions.

6. Explain the meaning of the 2 Trees in the garden and how it relates to your own choices.

7. What is the danger of your growing independence?

8. What did Adam and Eve do after they had eaten the forbidden fruit?

9. What can you learn from what Adam and Eve did after they sinned?

10. Explain why it is important to share your struggles with those adults whom you trust.

Total Health ·········· Chapter 1 • Quiz A Key

Unit 1: Physical Health   15 points

Section 1.1

MATCHING (5 points; 1 point each): For each numbered item, place the letter of the correct answer in the space provided at the left of each item. Each answer can be used only once.

1. __D__ Habits

2. __A__ Temptation

3. __C__ Influences

4. __E__ Deception

5. __B__ Consequences

A. Something that allures or draws you especially to evil.

B. The outcome or result of something.

C. Music, the media, church, friends, and your relationship with God.

D. Patterns of how you will handle life's challenges.

E. To trick or mislead someone.

SHORT ANSWER: (10 points; 2 points each) Answer the following questions.

6. Explain the meaning of the 2 Trees in the garden and how it relates to your own choices.

   The two trees represent the struggle between choosing God's truth—the tree of life, or choosing isolation, independence, and poor choices—the tree of death.

7. What is the danger of your growing independence?

   To think that you really don't need anyone in your life to help you through the struggles. Feeling like you should be able to handle all your problems on your own.

8. What did Adam and Eve do after they had eaten the forbidden fruit?

   They hid from God.

9. What can you learn from what Adam and Eve did after they sinned?

   God does not want you to hide from Him. He is waiting for you to come to Him, and share your struggles. He also will seek you out at times because He cares for you so much.

10. Explain why it is important to share your struggles with those adults whom you trust.

   God uses other people to help direct you and give you guidance and wisdom in your decisions. It will help you feel like you are not alone in your struggles if you talk to someone about them. Also, it gives you strength to overcome.

Total Health · Chapter 1 • Quiz B

Unit 1: Physical Health   Name:_____

Sections 1.2-1.3   Date: _____

15 Points   Score: _____

SHORT ANSWER: Answer the following questions.

1. What is meant by the term "soul"? (1 point)

2. Explain what is meant by the phrase "Total Health." (4 points)

3. How has Eve's decision affected all of mankind today? Give an example for each of the 4 categories. (4 points)

    Physical:

    Social:

    Mental:

    Spiritual:

4. Eve allowed Satan to entice her with his deceptive words and by the sight of delicious fruit. According to the following verses, how did Solomon advise people to handle evil influences? How might this truth apply to your daily life?

    My son, do not walk in the way with them, keep your foot from their path.
    Proverbs 1:15. (NKJ) (3 points)

    Do not be wise in your own eyes; fear the LORD and depart from evil.
    Proverbs 3:7. (NKJ) (3 points)

Total Health · Chapter 1 • Quiz B Key

Unit 1: Physical Health   15 points

Sections 1.2-1.3

SHORT ANSWER: Answer the following questions.

1. What is meant by the term "soul"? (1 point)
    Your mind, will, and emotions

2. Explain what is meant by the phrase "Total Health." (4 points)
    Total Health refers to all of those things that make up the whole person functioning well;
    physical, mental, social and spiritual.

3. How has Eve's decision affected all of mankind today? Give an example for each of the 4
    categories. (4 points)
    Physical: *disease, illness, death*

    Social: *conflict with others, jealousy*

    Mental: *struggle against nature, fear, stress*

    Spiritual: *separation from God*

4. Eve allowed Satan to entice her with his deceptive words and by the sight of delicious fruit.
    According to the following verses, how did Solomon advise people to handle evil influences?
    How might this truth apply to your daily life?

    My son, do not walk in the way with them, keep your foot from their path.
    Proverbs 1:15. (NKJ) (3 points)
    Keep from evil, don't even get close to those things that are not of God or bring temptation.

    Do not be wise in your own eyes; fear the LORD and depart from evil.
    Proverbs 3:7. (NKJ) (3 points)
    Have a healthy fear of God. Wanting to please a holy God will help keep you from evil.

Total Health ·············· Chapter 1 • Test

Unit 1: Physical Health

100 Points

Name:_____

Date: _____

Score: _____

MATCHING (18 points; 3 points each): For each numbered item, place the letter of the correct answer in the space provided at the left of each item. Each answer can be used only once.

1. _____ Habits

2. _____ Consequences

3. _____ Influences

4. _____ Temptation

5. _____ Deception

6. _____ Soul

A. To trick or mislead someone.

B. Music, the media, church, friends, and your relationship with God.

C. Patterns of how you will handle life's challenges.

D. The outcome or result of something.

E. A person's mind, will and emotions.

F. Something that allures or draws you especially to evil.

SHORT ANSWER: Answer the following questions.

7. What is the danger of your growing independence? (5 points)

8. What can you learn from what Adam and Eve did after they sinned? (5 points)

9. What did Adam and Eve do after they had eaten the forbidden fruit? (5 points)

10. Explain the meaning of the two Trees in the garden and how it relates to your own choices. (5 points)

11. Explain why it is important to share your struggles with those adults whom you trust. (5 points)

12. How has Eve's decision affected all of mankind today? Give an example for each of the 4 categories. (8 points)

    Physical: Social:

    Mental: Spiritual:

13. Explain what is meant by the phrase "Total Health." (7 points)

14. Fill in the four blanks in the Total Health wheel below which describe the four areas of life covered by the Total Health curriculum. (4 points)

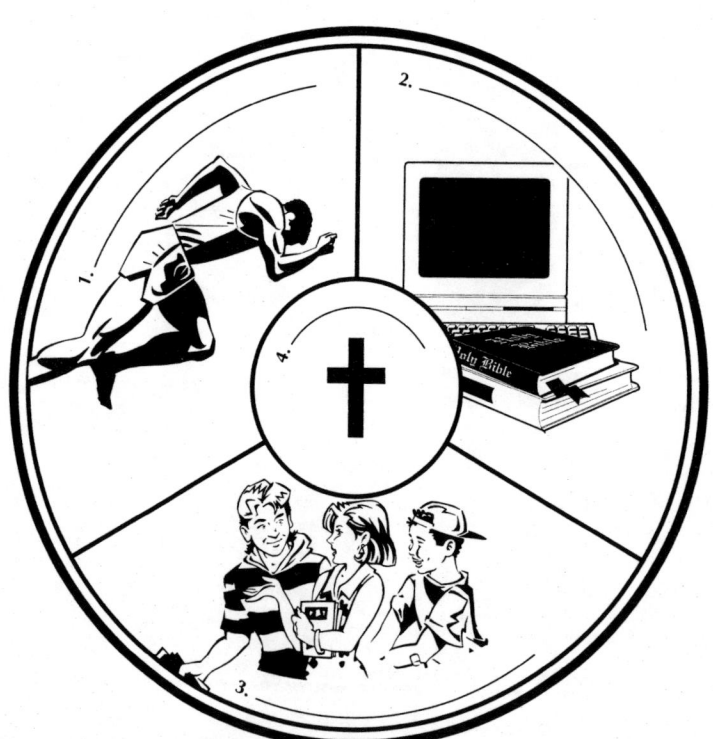

15. Fill in the key words left out of the following verse of I Thessalonians 5:23 which gives the scriptural basis for the Total Health concept: "Now may the God of peace Himself sanctify you completely; and may your whole _____, _____, and _____ be preserved blameless at the coming of our Lord Jesus Christ. He who calls you is faithful, who also will do it." (3 points)

16. When Adam and Eve ate from the forbidden tree, and hid from God, how did God respond to them? (4 points)

17. Evaluate yourself for a moment. Do you face your struggles alone, or do you talk to someone else about them? (3 points)

18. Who would be your first choice to talk to and why would you choose him/her? (4 points)

19. What makes him/her a positive or negative choice? (4 points)

ESSAY

20. What painful struggles might the "forbidden fruit" represent to you and many other young teenagers? (10 points)

(cont. ➤)

ESSAY

21. What choices do you face today that may positively or negatively influence your future? (10 points)

Total Health ································ Chapter 1 • Test Key

Unit 1: Physical Health   100 points

MATCHING (18 points; 3 points each): For each numbered item, place the letter of the correct answer in the space provided at the left of each item. Each answer can be used only once.

1. __C__ Habits
2. __D__ Consequences
3. __B__ Influences
4. __F__ Temptation
5. __A__ Deception
6. __E__ Soul

A. To trick or mislead someone.
B. Music, the media, church, friends, and your relationship with God.
C. Patterns of how you will handle life's challenges.
D. The outcome or result of something.
E. A person's mind, will and emotions.
F. Something that allures or draws you especially to evil.

SHORT ANSWER: Answer the following questions.

7. What is the danger of your growing independence? (5 points)

   To think that you really don't need anyone in your life to help you through the struggles. Feeling like you should be able to handle all your problems on your own.

8. What can you learn from what Adam and Eve did after they sinned? (5 points)

   God does not want you to hide from Him. He is waiting for you to come to Him, and share your struggles. He also will seek you out at times because He cares for you so much.

9. What did Adam and Eve do after they had eaten the forbidden fruit? (5 points)

   They hid from God.

10. Explain the meaning of the two Trees in the garden and how it relates to your own choices. (5 points)

    The two trees represent the struggle between choosing God's truth—the tree of life, or choosing isolation, independence, and poor choices—the tree of death.

11. Explain why it is important to share your struggles with those adults whom you trust. (5 points)

    God uses other people to help direct you and give you guidance and wisdom in your decisions. It will help you feel like you are not alone in your struggles if you talk to someone about them. Also, it gives you strength to overcome.

12. How has Eve's decision affected all of mankind today? Give an example for each of the 4 categories. (8 points)

    Physical: *disease, illness, death*   Social: *conflict with others, jealousy*

    Mental: *struggle against nature, fear, stress*   Spiritual: *separation from God*

13. Explain what is meant by the phrase "Total Health." (7 points)

    Total Health refers to all of those things that make up the whole person functioning well: physical, mental, social and spiritual.

14. Fill in the four blanks in the Total Health wheel below which describe the four areas of life covered by the Total Health curriculum. (4 points)

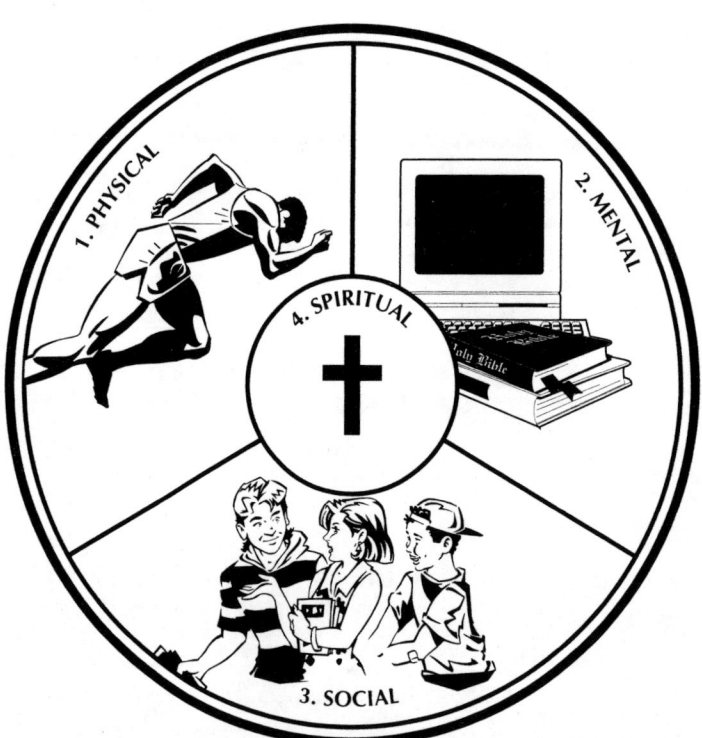

15. Fill in the key words left out of the following verse of I Thessalonians 5:23 which gives the scriptural basis for the Total Health concept: "Now may the God of peace Himself sanctify you completely; and may your whole _____*spirit*_____, _____*soul*_____, and _____*body*_____ be preserved blameless at the coming of our Lord Jesus Christ. He who calls you is faithful, who also will do it." (3 points)

16. When Adam and Eve ate from the forbidden tree, and hid from God, how did God respond to them? (4 points)

    He came and searched for them. He asked them where they were. He probed into their disobedience.

17. Evaluate yourself for a moment. Do you face your struggles alone, or do you talk to someone else about them? (3 points)

    Answers will vary. Hopefully, they talk with someone who they can trust.

18. Who would be your first choice to talk to and why would you choose him/her? (4 points)

    Answers will vary. They may choose their mom, dad, teacher, youth pastor, etc. The reason that they would choose him/her is because they can trust them, feel like they can open up to them and share, because they have a different perspective, feel like they could pray with them for strength.

19. What makes him/her a positive or negative choice? (4 points)

    Answers will vary. Could be somewhat of a personal repetition from the answer to the previous question.

ESSAY

20. What painful struggles might the "forbidden fruit" represent to you and many other young teenagers? (10 points)

    Answers will vary. They will probably include the negative sides of the following (taken from the text page 9):

    Media/entertainment: images of sex and violence, profanity, commercials ("You're not cool unless you buy this!"), magazines, advertisements, TV, computer/video games, star/celebrity lifestyles, the Internet, movies, videos.

    Music: lyrics, tunes, moods, sounds, MTV

    Friends: what you talk about, jokes, clothes, habits, what you do to have fun, comparing yourself with others, copying others

    Family: the tone in your voice, topics of conversation, daily habit patterns, good and bad examples

    Church: practical messages, relevant Bible studies, leaders who "walk the talk", feeling accepted as you are, finding genuine friends, having open discussions

    The Bible: reading and applying the Word of God to your daily struggles, how much you allow it to influence your life

    Relationship with God: how often you talk with Him, how much you want to follow Him, if you obey Him

ESSAY

21. What choices do you face today that may positively or negatively influence your future? (10 points)

    Answers will vary. They will probably include the points in the answer above worded in terms of a choice or a decision; both negatively and/or positively.

Total Health ····················· Chapter 2 • Quiz A

Unit 1: Physical Health

Sections 2.1-2.2

20 Points

Name:_____

Date: _____

Score: _____

MATCHING (8 points; 1 point each): For each numbered item, place the letter of the correct answer in the space provided at the left of each item. Each answer can be used only once.

1. _____ Healthy

2. _____ Cells

3. _____ Tissues

4. _____ Organ

A. The basic building blocks from which all larger parts are formed.

B. Your physical, mental, social and spiritual well-being.

C. Specialized groups within the body to carry out particular functions.

D. Example: your heart, kidneys, and lungs.

Match the types of tissues in the body with the letter of the correct example of that tissue.

5. _____ Connective tissue

6. _____ Epithelial tissue

7. _____ Muscle tissue

8. _____ Nerve tissue

A. Tendons, ligaments.

B. Skin.

C. Spinal cord, brain.

D. The heart.

SHORT ANSWER: Answer the following questions.

9. List the 8 common characteristics of single cells. (8 points)

   a.   e.

   b.   f.

   c.   g.

   d.   h.

10. List 4 things that can daily affect your body's state of health. (4 points)

Total Health .... Chapter 2 • Quiz A Key

Unit 1: Physical Health   20 points

Sections 2.1-2.2

MATCHING (8 points; 1 point each): For each numbered item, place the letter of the correct answer in the space provided at the left of each item. Each answer can be used only once.

1. __B__ Healthy

2. __A__ Cells

3. __C__ Tissues

4. __D__ Organ

A. The basic building blocks from which all larger parts are formed.

B. Your physical, mental, social and spiritual well-being.

C. Specialized groups within the body to carry out particular functions.

D. Example: your heart, kidneys, and lungs.

Match the types of tissues in the body with the letter of the correct example of that tissue.

5. __A__ Connective tissue   A. Tendons, ligaments.

6. __B__ Epithelial tissue   B. Skin.

7. __D__ Muscle tissue   C. Spinal cord, brain.

8. __C__ Nerve tissue   D. The heart.

SHORT ANSWER: Answer the following questions.

9. List the 8 common characteristics of single cells. (8 points)

   a. *moving*   e. *growing*

   b. *sensing*   f. *eliminating*

   c. *breathing*   g. *ingesting*

   d. *reproducing*   h. *living*

10. List 4 things that can daily affect your body's state of health. (4 points)

    stress, lack of sleep, food choices, exercise, exposure to germs, changes in the body

Total Health ·· Chapter 2 • Quiz B

Unit 1: Physical Health

Section 2.3 (Systems of the Body)

30 Points

Name:_____

Date: _____

Score: _____

MATCHING: (20 points; 1 point each) For each numbered item, place the letter of the correct answer in the space provided at the left of each item. Each answer can be used only once.

1.   _____ Pituitary gland

2.   _____ Alimentary canal

3.   _____ Blood pressure

4.   _____ Hormones

5.   _____ Red blood cells

6.   _____ Arteries

7.   _____ Small intestine

8.   _____ White blood cells

9.   _____ Epiglottis

10. _____ Homeostasis

11. _____ Large intestine

A. Carry oxygen through the blood.

B. Prevents food from entering the trachea.

C. The location where most of your digestion occurs.

D. Absorbs liquid and moves waste through the body.

E. A stable internal environment.

F. Carry blood filled with oxygen away from the heart.

G. Fight germs and viruses.

H. The force that your blood puts on the inside walls of your blood vessels.

I. Sometimes called "chemical messengers".

J. Often called the "master gland".

K. A long muscular tube that extends from the mouth to the anus.

Match the correct system with the letter of the correct definition or example of that system.

12. _____ Circulatory system

13. _____ Cardiovascular system

14. _____ Respiratory system

15. _____ Skeletal system

16. _____ Muscular system

17. _____ Digestive system

18. _____ Excretory system

19. _____ Nervous system

20. _____ Endocrine system

A. Multiple sclerosis is a disease that affects this system.

B. The kidneys are a part of this system.

C. This system is like a major road transportation network.

D. The heart.

E. The trachea is a part of this system.

F. Secretes hormones into your blood stream as messages to your cells.

G. Your alimentary canal.

H. This system works in pairs.

I. Arthritis affects this system.

SHORT ANSWER AND FILL IN THE BLANK: Answer the following questions.

21. Using arrows, draw the correct direction of blood flow through the heart. (2 points)

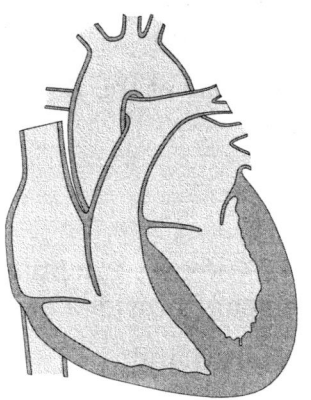

22. Label the following parts of the digestive system in the diagram: Esophagus, Liver, Stomach, Gall bladder, Small intestine. (5 points)

23. Which body systems are hurt by the poor eating habits a person might have? How does a poor diet hurt these systems? How might you change your personal diet to help these systems? (3 points)

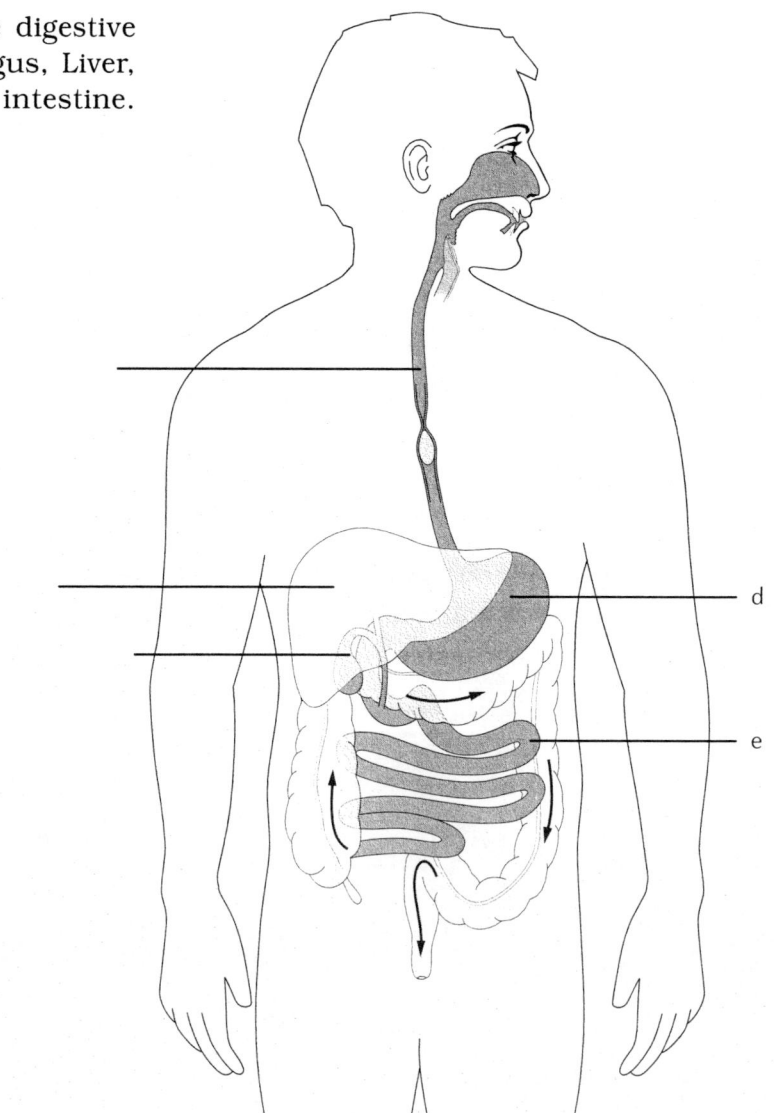

Total Health · Chapter 2 • Quiz B Key

Unit 1: Physical Health   30 points

Section 2.3 (Systems of the Body)

MATCHING: (20 points; 1 point each) For each numbered item, place the letter of the correct answer in the space provided at the left of each item. Each answer can be used only once.

1. _J_ Pituitary gland
2. _K_ Alimentary canal
3. _H_ Blood pressure
4. _I_ Hormones
5. _A_ Red blood cells
6. _F_ Arteries
7. _C_ Small intestine
8. _G_ White blood cells
9. _B_ Epiglottis
10. _E_ Homeostasis
11. _D_ Large intestine

A. Carry oxygen through the blood.
B. Prevents food from entering the trachea.
C. The location where most of your digestion occurs.
D. Absorbs liquid and moves waste through the body.
E. A stable internal environment.
F. Carry blood filled with oxygen away from the heart.
G. Fight germs and viruses.
H. The force that your blood puts on the inside walls of your blood vessels.
I. Sometimes called "chemical messengers".
J. Often called the "master gland".
K. A long muscular tube that extends from the mouth to the anus.

Match the correct system with the letter of the correct definition or example of that system.

12. _C_ Circulatory system
13. _D_ Cardiovascular system
14. _E_ Respiratory system
15. _I_ Skeletal system
16. _H_ Muscular system
17. _G_ Digestive system
18. _B_ Excretory system
19. _A_ Nervous system
20. _F_ Endocrine system

A. Multiple sclerosis is a disease that affects this system.
B. The kidneys are a part of this system.
C. This system is like a major road transportation network.
D. The heart.
E. The trachea is a part of this system.
F. Secretes hormones into your blood stream as messages to your cells.
G. Your alimentary canal.
H. This system works in pairs.
I. Arthritis affects this system.

SHORT ANSWER AND FILL IN THE BLANK: Answer the following questions.

21. Using arrows, draw the correct direction of blood flow through the heart. (2 points)

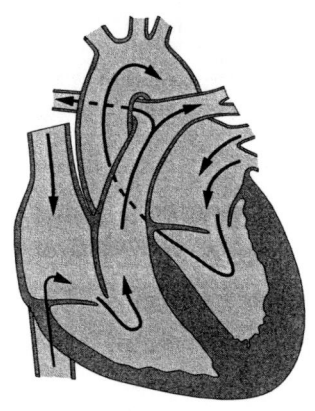

22. Label the following parts of the digestive system in the diagram: Esophagus, Liver, Stomach, Gall bladder, Small intestine. (5 points)

23. Which body systems are hurt by the poor eating habits a person might have? How does a poor diet hurt these systems? How might you change your personal diet to help these systems? (3 points)

Every body system is hurt by poor nutrition; however, the circulatory, cardiovascular, digestive, and excretory systems are more directly affected. Poor diet causes hardening of the arteries, lowers ability to fight off diseases, the heart must work harder than normal, the digestive system slows down and the excretory system becomes less efficient. Teens should consider less junk food that is high in salt, fat and sugar. Diet soda pop with the dangerous chemicals, as well as regular soda pop that is high in sugar should be limited in their diets. Eat more fresh vegetables and fruit to help these systems.

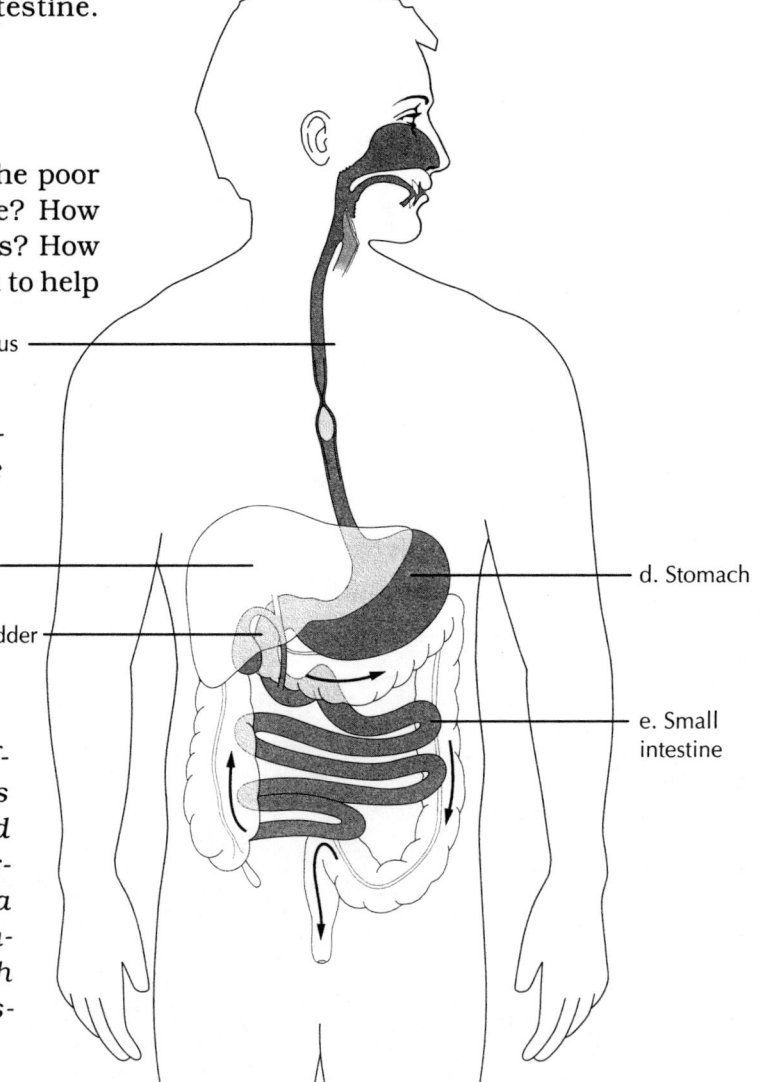

a. Esophagus

b. Liver

c. Gall bladder

d. Stomach

e. Small intestine

28

Total Health ···························· Chapter 2 • Test

Unit 1: Physical Health

100 Points

Name:_____

Date: _____

Score: _____

List the nine systems of the body, in any order, as taught in the student text. (9 points; 1 point each)

1.   6.

2.   7.

3.   8.

4.   9.

5.

MATCHING: (19 points; 1 point each) For each numbered item, place the letter of the correct answer in the space provided at the left of each item. Each answer can be used only once.

10. _____ Cells

11. _____ Tissues

12. _____ Organ

13. _____ Pituitary gland

14. _____ Alimentary canal

15. _____ Blood pressure

16. _____ Hormones

17. _____ Red blood cells

18. _____ Arteries

19. _____ Small intestine

20. _____ White blood cells

21. _____ Epiglottis

22. _____ Homeostasis

23. _____ Large intestine

A. Carry oxygen through the blood.

B. A stable internal environment.

C. The heart.

D. Carry blood filled with oxygen away from the heart.

E. Similar cells organized into specialized groups within the body to carry out particular functions.

F. The location where most of your digestion occurs.

G. Sometimes called "chemical messengers".

H. Absorbs liquid and moves waste through the body.

I. Prevents food from entering the trachea.

J. The force that your blood puts on the inside walls of your blood vessels.

K. The basic building blocks from which all larger parts are formed.

L. Often called the "master gland".

M. A long muscular tube that extends from the mouth to the anus.

N. Fight germs and viruses.

O. Examples: Liver, Kidneys, Heart.

Match the types of tissues in the body with the letter of the correct example of that tissue. (1 point each).

24. _____ Nerve tissue

25. _____ Epithelial tissue

26. _____ Muscle tissue

27. _____ Connective tissue

A. Cause body parts to move.

B. Skin.

C. Tendons, ligaments.

D. Receive and transmit impulses to the brain.

29

SHORT ANSWER: Answer the following questions.

28. Which body systems are hurt by the poor eating habits a person might have? (5 points)

29. How does a poor diet hurt these systems? (5 points)

30. How might you change your personal diet to help these systems? (5 points)

31. List four things that can daily affect your body's state of health. (8 points; 2 points each)

32. List four facts or observations about your body that show how awesome of a creation it is. (4 points)

33. List the 8 common characteristics of single cells. (8 points; 1 point each)

   a.   e.

   b.   f.

   c.   g.

   d.   h.

34. Using arrows, draw the correct direction of blood flow through the heart in the diagram below. Also, explain what is happening at each step. (12 points; 2 points each)

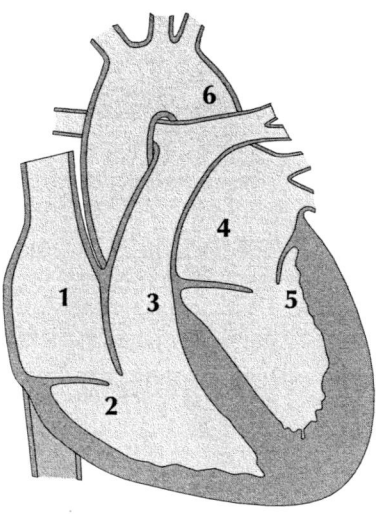

35. Label the ten parts of the digestive and excretory systems in the diagram below. (10 points; 1 point each)

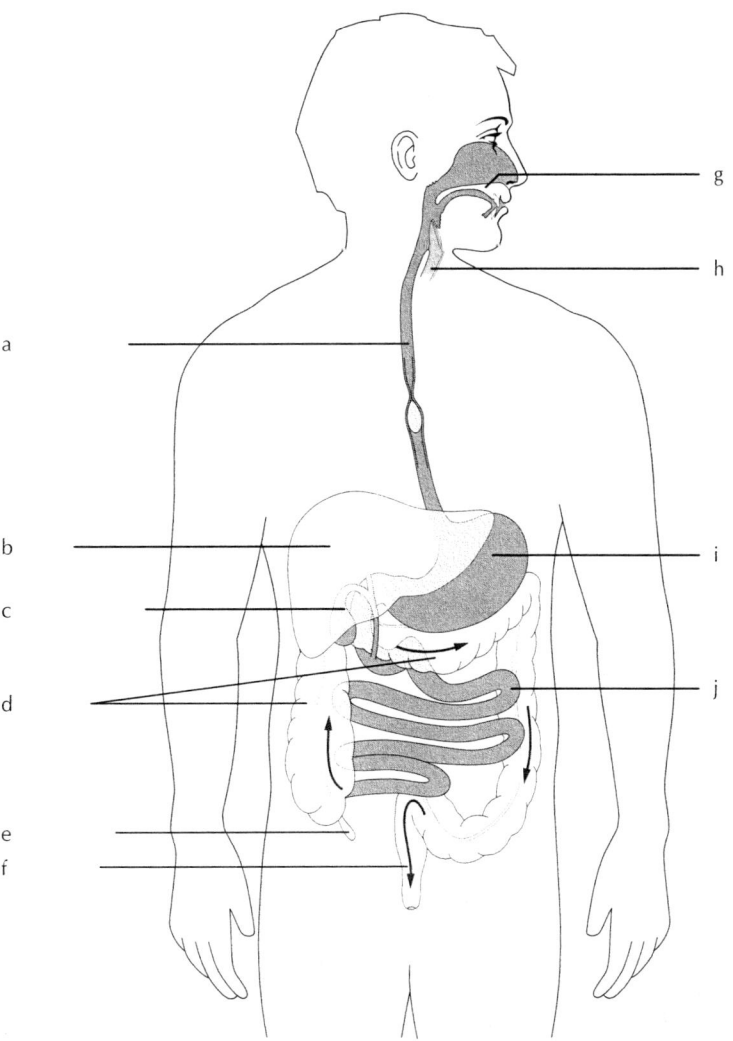

ESSAY (11 points)

36. What body systems are helped by consistent physical activity? How does exercise help them? In what ways might you change your physical exercise routine?

"I would change my exercise routine by..."

Total Health ············· Chapter 2 • Test Key

Unit 1: Physical Health   100 points

List the nine systems of the body, in any order, as taught in the student text. (9 points; 1 point each)

1. *Circulatory*   6. *Excretory*
2. *Respiratory*   7. *Endocrine*
3. *Skeletal*   8. *Nervous*
4. *Muscular*   9. *Cardiovascular*
5. *Digestive*

MATCHING: (19 points; 1 point each) For each numbered item, place the letter of the correct answer in the space provided at the left of each item. Each answer can be used only once.

10. _K_ Cells
11. _E_ Tissues
12. _O_ Organ
13. _L_ Pituitary gland
14. _M_ Alimentary canal
15. _J_ Blood pressure
16. _G_ Hormones
17. _A_ Red blood cells
18. _D_ Arteries
19. _F_ Small intestine
20. _N_ White blood cells
21. _I_ Epiglottis
22. _B_ Homeostasis
23. _H_ Large intestine

A. Carry oxygen through the blood.
B. A stable internal environment.
C. The heart.
D. Carry blood filled with oxygen away from the heart.
E. Similar cells organized into specialized groups within the body to carry out particular functions.
F. The location where most of your digestion occurs.
G. Sometimes called "chemical messengers".
H. Absorbs liquid and moves waste through the body.
I. Prevents food from entering the trachea.
J. The force that your blood puts on the inside walls of your blood vessels.
K. The basic building blocks from which all larger parts are formed.
L. Often called the "master gland".
M. A long muscular tube that extends from the mouth to the anus.
N. Fight germs and viruses.
O. Examples: Liver, Kidneys, Heart.

Match the types of tissues in the body with the letter of the correct example of that tissue. (1 point each).

24. _D_ Nerve tissue
25. _B_ Epithelial tissue
26. _A_ Muscle tissue
27. _C_ Connective tissue

A. Cause body parts to move.
B. Skin.
C. Tendons, ligaments.
D. Receive and transmit impulses to the brain.

SHORT ANSWER: Answer the following questions.

28. Which body systems are hurt by the poor eating habits a person might have? (5 points)

    Every body system is hurt by poor nutrition; however, the circulatory, cardiovascular, digestive, and excretory systems are more directly affected.

29. How does a poor diet hurt these systems? (5 points)

    Poor diet causes hardening of the arteries, lowers ability to fight off diseases, the heart must work harder than normal, the digestive system slows down and the excretory system becomes less efficient.

30. How might you change your personal diet to help these systems? (5 points)

    Teens should consider less junk food that is high in salt, fat and sugar. Diet soda pop with the dangerous chemicals, as well as regular soda pop that is high in sugar should be limited in their diets. Eat more fresh vegetables and fruit to help these systems.

31. List four things that can daily affect your body's state of health. (8 points; 2 points each)

    stress, lack of sleep, food choices, exercise, exposure to germs, changes in the body

32. List four facts or observations about your body that show how awesome of a creation it is. (4 points)

    The body is made to heal itself, regenerate cells, its skin changing and growing, the awesome function of the eyes and ears.

33. List the 8 common characteristics of single cells. (8 points; 1 point each)

    a. *moving*   e. *growing*
    b. *sensing*   f. *eliminating*
    c. *breathing*   g. *ingesting*
    d. *reproducing*   h. *living*

34. Using arrows, draw the correct direction of blood flow through the heart in the diagram below. Also, explain what is happening at each step. (12 points; 2 points each)

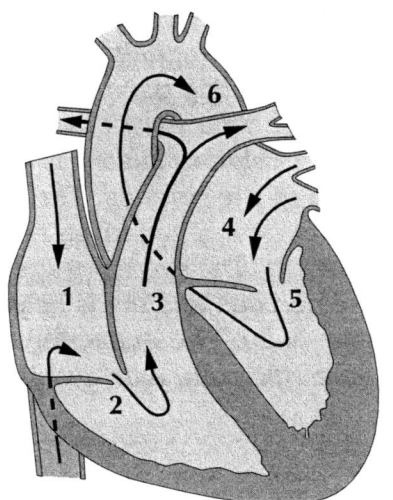

1. *Blood from body enters right atrium through superior vena cava and inferior vena cava.*

2. *Blood enters right ventricle through tricuspid valve.*

3. *Heart pumps blood from right ventricle to pulmonary trunk, which carries blood to the lungs where oxygen is absorbed.*

4. *Blood carrying oxygen is returned to the left atrium through the pulmonary veins.*

5. *Blood enters left ventricle through bicuspid valve.*

6. *Heart pumps blood from left ventricle to aorta, which carries blood to the body.*

35. Label the ten parts of the digestive and excretory systems in the diagram below. (10 points; 1 point each)

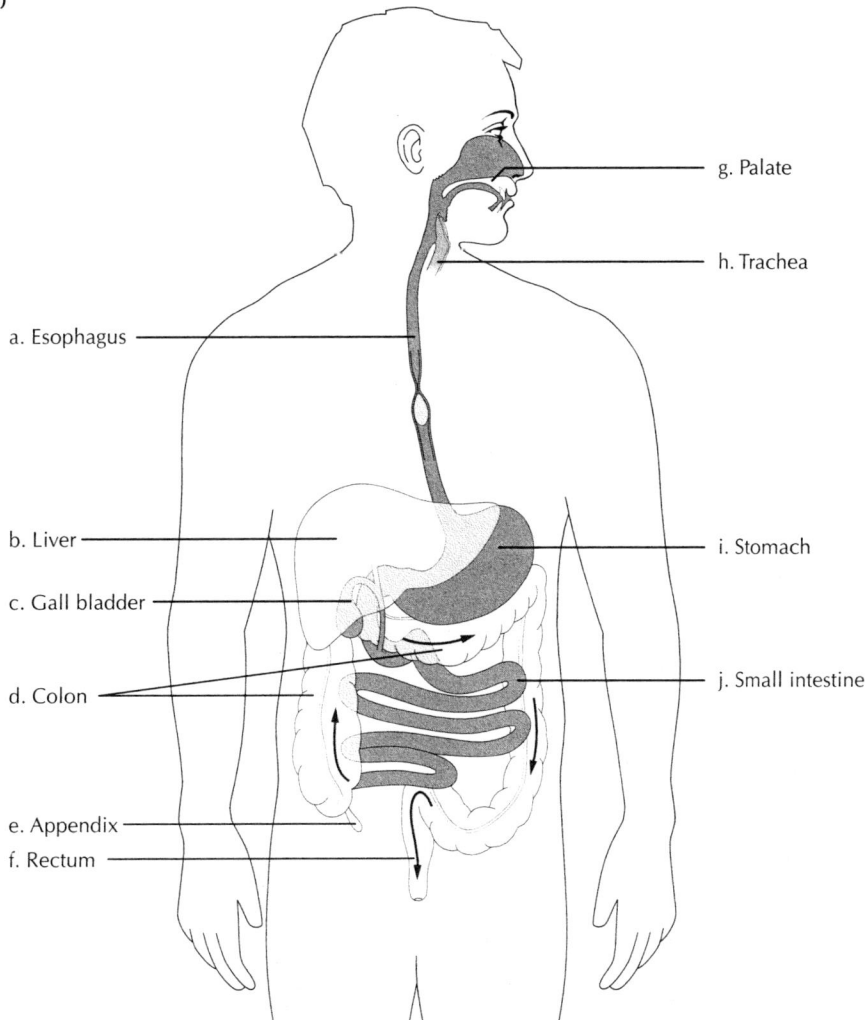

g. Palate

h. Trachea

a. Esophagus

b. Liver

c. Gall bladder

d. Colon

e. Appendix

f. Rectum

i. Stomach

j. Small intestine

ESSAY (11 points)

36. What body systems are helped by consistent physical activity? How does exercise help them? In what ways might you change your physical exercise routine?

    All systems are helped by consistent physical activity. The bones and muscles are strengthened, enabling you to withstand more physical activity, stand up straighter, and have more stamina. Your heart, which is the most important muscle of the body, is strengthened while your circulatory system is kept cleansed, helping to prevent cardiovascular disease and hardening of the arteries. The respiratory system brings vital oxygen to the circulatory system and is strengthened by activity. The digestive system is better able to digest and absorb nutrients. The excretory system stays cleansed by exercise promoting the movement of waste. The nervous system is helped because exercise helps to release stress that can build up in your body. The endocrine systems are also strengthened because the whole body works more efficiently with consistent exercise.

    "I would change my exercise routine by..."
    Answers may vary.

Total Health · Chapter 3 • Quiz A

Unit 1: Physical Health   Name:_____

Section 3.1   Date: _____

20 Points   Score: _____

DEFINE (5 points; 1 point each): Define the following terms as they are defined in the text.

1. Balanced diet:

2. Empty calories:

3. Nutrients:

4. Vegetarian diet:

5. Calories:

MATCHING (6 points; 1 point each): For each numbered item, place the letter of the correct answer in the space provided at the left of each item. Each answer can be used only once.

6. _____ Proteins
7. _____ Carbohydrates
8. _____ Fats
9. _____ Cholesterol
10. _____ Saturated fat
11. _____ Unsaturated fat

A. What is left in the pan after frying a piece of hamburger meat.

B. Sugars and starches.

C. Builds new cell tissue.

D. Concentrated source of energy.

E. Liquid at room temperature and does not tend to raise cholesterol levels.

F. A fatty substance in the blood which increases the risk of heart disease.

SHORT ANSWER: Answer the following questions.

12. Explain how a pizza could be a potentially healthy meal. With this in mind, describe what kind of "healthy" pizza you would order. (4 points)

13. Explain why it is a good idea not to drink a liquid while you are eating your meal. (1 point)

14. Explain why your body needs an adequate amount of water each day. Include in your answer how much water a person should drink in a day and 3 of the 6 ways your body uses water. (4 points)

Total Health ································· Chapter 3 • Quiz A Key

Unit 1: Physical Health   20 points

Section 3.1

DEFINE (5 points; 1 point each): Define the following terms as they are defined in the text.

1. Balanced diet: *making food choices that include a wide variety from all that God has given to us in nature.*

2. Empty calories: *those foods that don't have any nutritive value.*

3. Nutrients: *substances in foods that your body needs (proteins, carbohydrates, fats, vitamins, minerals and water).*

4. Vegetarian diet: *a diet that typically excludes animal products.*

5. Calories: *a unit of heat that your body uses for activity*

MATCHING (6 points; 1 point each): For each numbered item, place the letter of the correct answer in the space provided at the left of each item. Each answer can be used only once.

6. _C_ Proteins
7. _B_ Carbohydrates
8. _D_ Fats
9. _F_ Cholesterol
10. _A_ Saturated fat
11. _E_ Unsaturated fat

A. What is left in the pan after frying a piece of hamburger meat.
B. Sugars and starches.
C. Builds new cell tissue.
D. Concentrated source of energy.
E. Liquid at room temperature and does not tend to raise cholesterol levels.
F. A fatty substance in the blood which increases the risk of heart disease.

SHORT ANSWER: Answer the following questions.

12. Explain how a pizza could be a potentially healthy meal. With this in mind, describe what kind of "healthy" pizza you would order. (4 points)

A pizza contains carbohydrates, vegetables, and protein. A healthy pizza order would include: low-fat cheeses, whole-wheat crust, and be topped with lots of vegetables.

13. Explain why it is a good idea not to drink a liquid while you are eating your meal. (1 point)

    It dilutes the digestive enzymes needed to begin the digestion process of your meal.

14. Explain why your body needs an adequate amount of water each day. Include in your answer how much water a person should drink in a day and 3 of the 6 ways your body uses water. (4 points)

    Water is the most common nutrient in your body. Without water you would die. Your body uses water for cleansing of waste and toxins, lubricating joints, transporting nutrients, regulating body temperature, losing weight, and digesting food.

Total Health ·················· Chapter 3 • Quiz B

Unit 1: Physical Health

Sections 3.2-3.3

20 Points

Name:_____

Date: _____

Score: _____

TRUE OR FALSE: (12 points; 2 points each) If the answer is true, put a T in the space provided. If the answer is false, put an F in the space provided. If the answer is false, write in the correct answer to make it true.

1. _____ Yo-yo dieting reduces your metabolic rate.

2. _____ Teens who are obese are more than 20% over their ideal weight.

3. _____ Anorexia is a pattern of "bingeing" and "purging".

4. _____ Bulimia is "self starvation".

5. _____ Chronic over-eating is more common than anorexia or bulimia among teens.

6. _____ Being overweight means weighing more than the desired weight for your age, height, sex and frame size.

SHORT ANSWER: Answer the following questions.

7. Explain what is meant by the phrase, "Junk food damages your body at the cellular level". (1 point)

8. When do healthy food choices begin to make a positive difference with your health? (1 point)

9. How might you change or adjust the Food Pyramid to be even healthier than it is? (1 point)

10. Explain 3 dangers of "fad" diets. (3 points)

   a.

   b.

   c.

11. List 2 of the 5 steps to remember when reading product labels. (2 points)

   a.

   b.

Total Health ··· **Chapter 3 • Quiz B Key**

Unit 1: Physical Health   20 points

Sections 3.2-3.3

TRUE OR FALSE: (12 points; 2 points each) If the answer is true, put a T in the space provided. If the answer is false, put an F in the space provided. If the answer is false, write in the correct answer to make it true.

1. _T_ Yo-yo dieting reduces your metabolic rate.

2. _T_ Teens who are obese are more than 20% over their ideal weight.

3. _F_ Anorexia is a pattern of "bingeing" and "purging". *bulimia*

4. _F_ Bulimia is "self starvation". *anorexia*

5. _T_ Chronic over-eating is more common than anorexia or bulimia among teens.

6. _T_ Being overweight means weighing more than the desired weight for your age, height, sex and frame size.

SHORT ANSWER: Answer the following questions.

7. Explain what is meant by the phrase, "Junk food damages your body at the cellular level". (1 point)

    All life begins at the smallest cellular level in your body. The health of the cells make up the tissues, the health of the tissues make up the health of your body systems and your health. Your cells take in nutrients for the whole body.

8. When do healthy food choices begin to make a positive difference with your health? (1 point)
    Right now!

9. How might you change or adjust the Food Pyramid to be even healthier than it is? (1 point)
    vegetables and fruit on the bottom

10. Explain 3 dangers of "fad" diets. (3 points)
    a. *They make promises that are unhealthy, i.e., quick weight loss makes you think of the short-term.*

    b. *Most of them have lots of sugar or artificial sweeteners.*

    c. *Most of them lack vital nutrients/minerals.*

11. List 2 of the 5 steps to remember when reading product labels. (2 points)
    a. *Do not be swayed by packaging.*

    b. *Check serving size, saturated fats, cholesterol, carbs-to-protein ratio, and oils.*

43

Total Health ································· Chapter 3 • Test

Unit 1: Physical Health

100 Points

Name:_____

Date: _____

Score: _____

MATCHING (12 points; 2 points each): For each numbered item, place the letter of the correct answer in the space provided at the left of each item. Each answer can be used only once.

1. ____ Proteins

2. ____ Carbohydrates

3. ____ Fats

4. ____ Cholesterol

5. ____ Saturated fat

6. ____ Unsaturated fat

A. Sugars and starches.

B. Concentrated source of energy.

C. Builds new cell tissue.

D. What is left in the pan after frying a piece of hamburger meat.

E. A fatty substance in the blood which increases the risk of heart disease.

F. Liquid at room temperature and do not tend to raise cholesterol levels.

SHORT ANSWER

7. Explain why your body needs an adequate amount of water each day. (3 points)

8. How much water should a person drink each day? (2 points)

9. What are 3 of the 6 ways your body uses water? (6 points; 2 points each)

DEFINE (10 points; 2 points each): Define the following terms as they are defined in the text.

10. Balanced diet:

11. Empty calories:

12. Nutrients:

13. Vegetarian diet:

14. Calories:

TRUE OR FALSE: (12 points; 2 points each) If the answer is true, put a T in the space provided. If the answer is false, put an F in the space provided. If the answer is false, write in the correct answer to make it true.

15. _____ Anorexia is "self starvation".

16. _____ Teens who are "obese" are more than 35% over their ideal weight.

17. _____ Chronic over-eating is a pattern of "bingeing" and "purging".

18. _____ Yo-yo dieting reduces your metabolic rate.

19. _____ Studies show that being "overweight" as a young person makes it more difficult to reach and maintain your ideal weight as an adult.

20. _____ If you want to help people who are suffering from an eating disorder, you should never eat around them.

SHORT ANSWER: Answer the following questions.

21. Explain how a pizza could be a potentially healthy meal. (3 points)

22. With this in mind, describe what kind of "healthy" pizza you would order. (5 points)

23. When do healthy food choices begin to make a positive difference with your health? (3 points)

24. Explain what is meant by the phrase, "Junk food damages your body at the cellular level". (5 points)

25. Explain 3 dangers of "fad" diets. (6 points; 2 points each)
    a.

    b.

    c.

26. Label the following Food Pyramid with the correct food groups. Include the number of servings suggested for each group. (12 points)

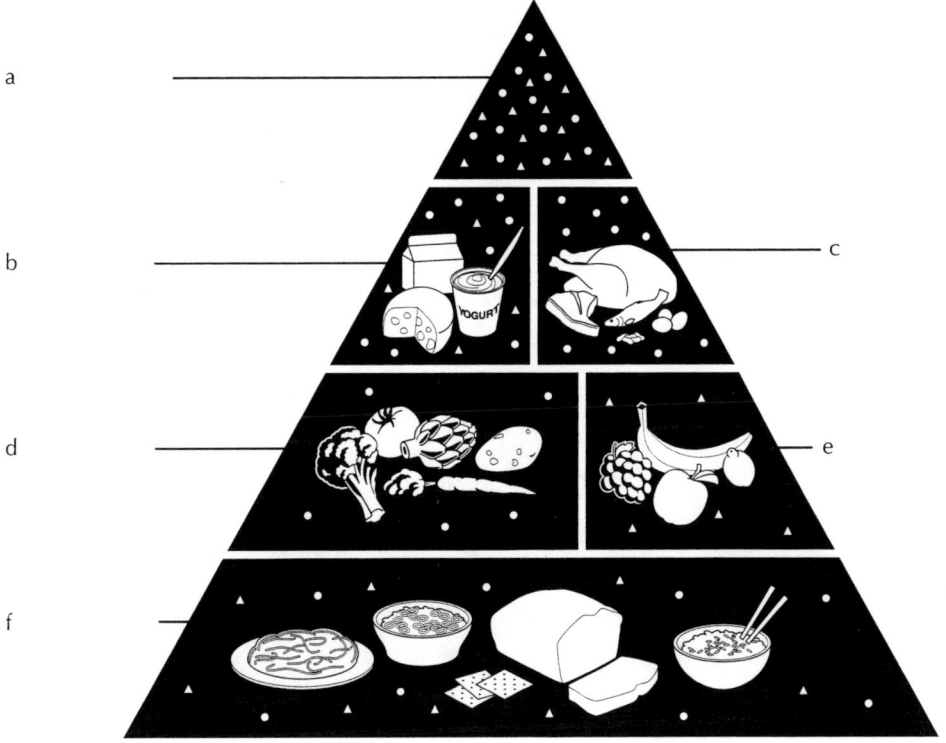

27. How might you change or adjust the Food Pyramid to be even healthier than it is? (4 points)

28. How you might benefit from keeping a food journal? (2 points)

ESSAY

29. Imagine that you have a friend(s) about whose poor eating habits you are very concerned. How might you determine if they have a problem with anorexia? How might you determine if they have a problem with bulimia? What might you say and/or do to help your friend? (15 points) *Use back of this page to complete your essay.*

Total Health · Chapter 3 • Test Key

Unit 1: Physical Health   100 points

MATCHING (12 points; 2 points each): For each numbered item, place the letter of the correct answer in the space provided at the left of each item. Each answer can be used only once.

1. _C_ Proteins
2. _A_ Carbohydrates
3. _B_ Fats
4. _E_ Cholesterol
5. _D_ Saturated fat
6. _F_ Unsaturated fat

A. Sugars and starches.
B. Concentrated source of energy.
C. Builds new cell tissue.
D. What is left in the pan after frying a piece of hamburger meat.
E. A fatty substance in the blood which increases the risk of heart disease.
F. Liquid at room temperature and do not tend to raise cholesterol levels.

SHORT ANSWER

7. Explain why your body needs an adequate amount of water each day. (3 points)
   Water is the most common nutrient in your body. Without water you would die.

8. How much water should a person drink each day? (2 points)
   At least 7-10 eight oz. glasses per day.

9. What are 3 of the 6 ways your body uses water? (6 points; 2 points each)
   Your body uses water for cleansing of waste and toxins, lubricating joints, transporting nutrients, regulating body temperature, losing weight, and digesting food.

DEFINE (10 points; 2 points each): Define the following terms as they are defined in the text.

10. Balanced diet: *making food choices that include a wide variety from all that God has given to us in nature.*

11. Empty calories: *those foods that don't have any nutritive value.*

12. Nutrients: *substances in foods that your body needs (proteins, carbohydrates, fats, vitamins, minerals and water).*

13. Vegetarian diet: *a diet that typically excludes animal products.*

14. Calories: *a unit of heat that your body uses for activity.*

49

TRUE OR FALSE: (12 points; 2 points each) If the answer is true, put a T in the space provided. If the answer is false, put an F in the space provided. If the answer is false, write in the correct answer to make it true.

15. __T__ Anorexia is "self starvation".

16. __F__ Teens who are "obese" are more than 35% over their ideal weight.
    20%

17. __F__ Chronic over-eating is a pattern of "bingeing" and "purging".
    Bulimia is.

18. __T__ Yo-yo dieting reduces your metabolic rate.

19. __T__ Studies show that being "overweight" as a young person makes it more difficult to reach and maintain your ideal weight as an adult.

20. __F__ If you want to help people who are suffering from an eating disorder, you should never eat around them.
    Help by acting normal around them

SHORT ANSWER: Answer the following questions.

21. Explain how a pizza could be a potentially healthy meal. (3 points)
    A pizza contains carbohydrates, vegetables, and protein.

22. With this in mind, describe what kind of "healthy" pizza you would order. (5 points)
    A healthy pizza order would include: low-fat cheeses, whole-wheat crust and topped with lots of vegetables.

23. When do healthy food choices begin to make a positive difference with your health? (3 points)
    Right now! Right away!

24. Explain what is meant by the phrase, "Junk food damages your body at the cellular level". (5 points) *All life begins at the smallest cellular level in your body. The health of the cells make up the tissues, the health of the tissues make up the health of your body systems and your health. Your cells take in nutrients for the whole body.*

25. Explain 3 dangers of "fad" diets. (6 points; 2 points each)
    a. *They make promises that are unhealthy, i.e., quick weight loss makes you think of the short-term.*
    b. *Most of them have lots of sugar or artificial sweeteners.*
    c. *Most of them lack vital nutrients/minerals.*

26. Label the following Food Pyramid with the correct food groups. Include the number of servings suggested for each group. (12 points)

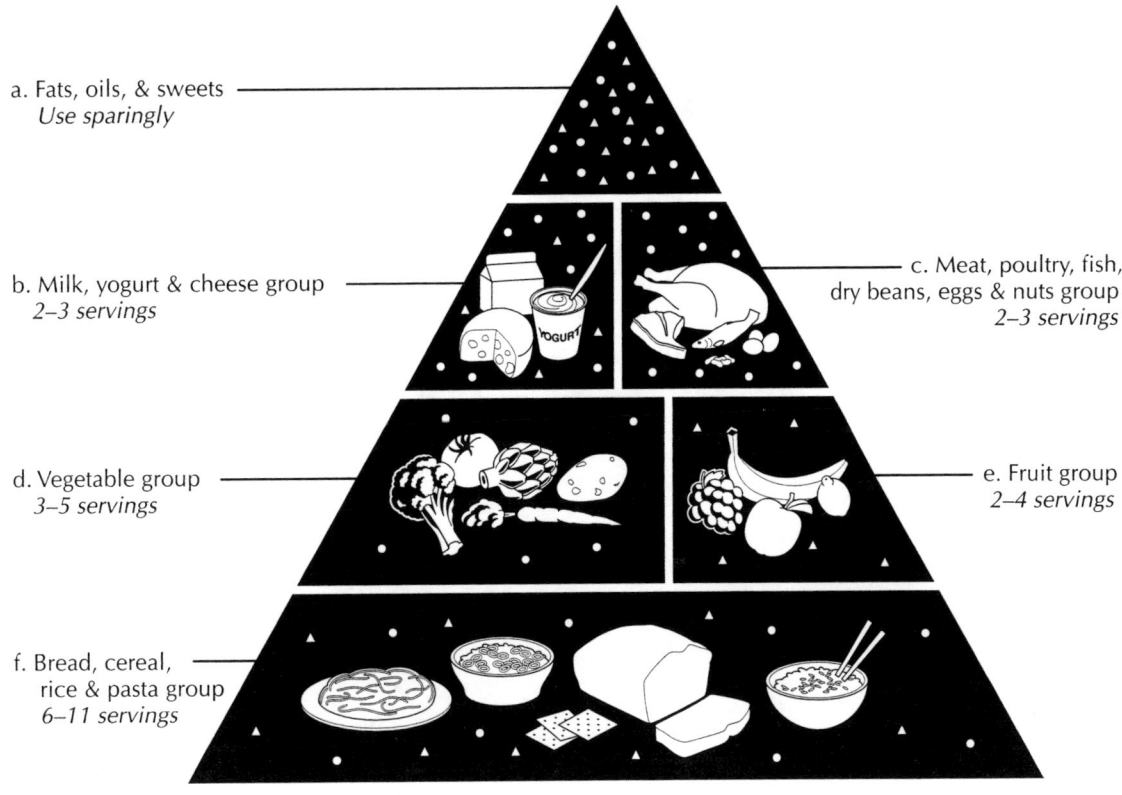

a. Fats, oils, & sweets
   Use sparingly

b. Milk, yogurt & cheese group
   2–3 servings

c. Meat, poultry, fish, dry beans, eggs & nuts group
   2–3 servings

d. Vegetable group
   3–5 servings

e. Fruit group
   2–4 servings

f. Bread, cereal, rice & pasta group
   6–11 servings

27. How might you change or adjust the Food Pyramid to be even healthier than it is? (4 points)
   Put the vegetables and fruit on the bottom of the pyramid instead of the grains.

28. How you might benefit from keeping a food journal? (2 points)
   Helps you find unhealthy patterns or weaknesses in your eating habits.

   Filling in the comment section helps you to understand details of your eating patterns with statements like, "I ate cookies when I was angry at my Mom," or "I got a headache after I ate that soda and chocolate candy."

ESSAY

29. Imagine that you have a friend(s) about whose poor eating habits you are very concerned. How might you determine if they have a problem with anorexia? How might you determine if they have a problem with bulimia? What might you say and/or do to help your friend? (15 points) *Use back of this page to complete your essay.*

   Signs of Anorexia:
   • *If they feel that they should lose weight even though they don't really have to.*
   • *If they don't eat a proper amount of food to maintain good health.*

51

- *If they show signs of wanting to have the "perfect" body.*

Signs of Bulimia:
- *If they have a habit of eating large portions of food and then vomiting it up on purpose (binging and purging).*
- *If they always go to the bathroom after eating a large meal.*

Answers should include some of the following:
- *Encourage them to talk about their feelings to an adult they trust.*
- *Don't nag them about their food.*
- *Help them to realize that it's normal to experience times in their lives when they spend extra effort and energy trying to accomplish something.*
- *Be there for them, especially if their parents don't understand their highs and lows.*
- *Show them love and acceptance as people—just as they are—with no strings attached.*

Total Health ·································· Chapter 4 • Quiz A

Unit 1: Physical Health   Name:_____

Sections 4.1-4.2   Date: _____

20 Points   Score: _____

DEFINE: (5 points; 1 point each) Define the following terms as they are defined in the text.

1. Fitness:

2. Cardiovascular fitness:

3. Aerobic:

4. Anaerobic:

5. Atrophy:

SHORT ANSWER: Answer the following questions.

6. Explain why the most important measurement of your fitness is cardiovascular fitness. (1 point)

7. List 6 benefits of exercise. (6 points; 1 point each) (more answers on page 80 in student text)
   - a.
   - b.
   - c.
   - d.
   - e.
   - f.

8. Explain 5 reasons why your joint muscle flexibility is important. (5 points)
   - a.
   - b.
   - c.
   - d.
   - e.

9. What is meant by the term "body composition"? Give 2 benefits to increasing your lean muscle weight. (3 points)

   Body composition is:

   Two benefits of increasing your lean muscle weight are:
   - a.
   - b.

Total Health ······················ **Chapter 4 • Quiz A Key**

Unit 1: Physical Health   20 points

Sections 4.1-4.2

DEFINE: (5 points; 1 point each) Define the following terms as they are defined in the text.

1. Fitness: *the ability of your mind and body to work together to their highest possible level*

2. Cardiovascular fitness: *the condition of the heart*

3. Aerobic: *when your muscles demand more oxygen than normal during exercise*

4. Anaerobic: *short bursts of activity without the use of much oxygen*

5. Atrophy: *when a long period of time lapses between workouts and the muscles decrease in size and strength*

SHORT ANSWER: Answer the following questions.

6. Explain why the most important measurement of your fitness is cardiovascular fitness. (1 point)
   A strong heart, along with healthy lungs and blood vessels, work together to supply oxygenated blood to the whole body. Without good cardiovascular fitness, it would not matter how much weight you could lift if you died from a heart attack!

7. List 6 benefits of exercise. (6 points; 1 point each) (more answers on page 80 in student text)
   a. *increases strength, stamina*   d. *relieves depression*
   b. *reduces stress, tension*   e. *reduces body fat*
   c. *improves mental alertness*   f. *increases BMR*

8. Explain 5 reasons why your joint muscle flexibility is important. (5 points)
   a. *reduces chance of injury*   d. *helps clear the mind*
   b. *helps coordination*   e. *improves circulation*
   c. *makes you feel better, reduces tension, makes work easier*

9. What is meant by the term "body composition"? Give 2 benefits to increasing your lean muscle weight. (3 points)
   Body composition is: *the relationship between your fat and lean (muscle) body weight.*

   Two benefits of increasing your lean muscle weight are:
   a. *burns more calories while you are at rest*
   b. *decreases your body fat*

Total Health · Chapter 4 • Quiz B

Unit 1: Physical Health

Sections 4.3-4.5

25 Points

Name:_____

Date: _____

Score: _____

TRUE OR FALSE: (12 points; 2 points each) If the answer is true, put a T in the space provided. If the answer is false, put an F in the space provided. If the answer is false, write in the correct answer to make it true.

1. _____ The first step in a proper warm-up is thoroughly stretching you muscles.

2. _____ The warm-up should last anywhere between 8–15 minutes.

3. _____ A warm-down consists of a slow jog or walk with some stretching.

4. _____ A warm-up or warm-down will help prevent injuries.

5. _____ Your body as a teenager is indestructible.

6. _____ When injured, the first thing to do is to get heat on the injury.

SHORT ANSWER: Answer the following questions.

7. Explain what is meant by the phrase, "accidental workout". Include in your answer any accidental workouts that your personal life already includes. (3 points)

8. Explain what is meant by the term "lifetime sports". List 3 examples of lifetime sports. (4 points)

   • Lifetime sports are:

   • 3 examples include:

9. Many teens compare themselves with others. How can comparison be dangerous and what does God think about it? (2 points)

10. Explain each step in the treatment of injuries following the acronym R.I.C.E. (4 points)

Total Health · Chapter 4 • Quiz B Key

Unit 1: Physical Health   25 points

Sections 4.3-4.5

TRUE OR FALSE: (12 points; 2 points each) If the answer is true, put a T in the space provided. If the answer is false, put an F in the space provided. If the answer is false, write in the correct answer to make it true.

1. __F__ The first step in a proper warm-up is thoroughly stretching you muscles.
   light movement, large muscle groups

2. __T__ The warm-up should last anywhere between 8–15 minutes.

3. __T__ A warm-down consists of a slow jog or walk with some stretching.

4. __T__ A warm-up or warm-down will help prevent injuries.

5. __F__ Your body as a teenager is indestructible.
   No way! You can get hurt.

6. __F__ When injured, the first thing to do is to get heat on the injury.
   Ice

SHORT ANSWER: Answer the following questions.

7. Explain what is meant by the phrase, "accidental workout". Include in your answer any accidental workouts that your personal life already includes. (3 points)

   An accidental workout means to increase your activity level when you don't even know you are doing it. It is making exercise and movement a fun and enjoyable part of your daily life. E.g., riding horses, bike riding, skateboarding, jump rope, etc.

8. Explain what is meant by the term "lifetime sports". List 3 examples of lifetime sports. (4 points)

   • Lifetime sports are: *activities that a person can participate in throughout a lifetime*

   • 3 examples include: *tennis, walking, golf, jogging*

9. Many teens compare themselves with others. How can comparison be dangerous and what does God think about it? (2 points)

   Comparing with your peers concerning appearance and skill. Comparing is one of the greatest enemies to your mind because it will either make you feel superior to others who aren't as good as you, or make you feel inferior to others who are better than you. God never intended for you to compare yourself with others. God only expects you to do your best and become the finest person you can become with the resources He's given to you.

10. Explain each step in the treatment of injuries following the acronym R.I.C.E. (4 points)
    Rest, Ice, Compression, Elevate

Total Health · Chapter 4 • Test

Unit 1: Physical Health

100 Points

Name:_____

Date: _____

Score: _____

DEFINE: Define the following terms as they are defined in the text. (14 points; 2 points each)

1. Anaerobic:

2. Fitness:

3. Aerobic:

4. Atrophy:

5. Cardiovascular fitness:

6. Muscular fitness:

7. Flexibility:

SHORT ANSWER: Answer the following questions.

8. Explain what is meant by the phrase, "accidental workout". Include in your answer any accidental workouts that your personal life includes already. (3 points)

9. List 6 benefits of exercise. (12 points; 2 points each)

    a.   d.

    b.   e.

    c.   f.

10. List 5 reasons why your joint muscle flexibility is important. (5 points; 1 point each)

    a.   d.

    b.   e.

    c.

11. List each step in the treatment of injuries following the acronym R.I.C.E. (4 points; 1 point each)

12. Explain what is meant by the term "body composition"? (3 points)
    Body composition is:

13. Give 2 benefits to increasing your lean muscle weight. (4 points; 2 points each)
    Two benefits of increasing my lean muscle weight are:
    a.

    b.

14. Explain why the phrase, "No pain, No gain" is incorrect when it comes to stretching and exercise? (4 points)

TRUE OR FALSE: (12 points; 2 points each) If the answer is true, put a T in the space provided. If the answer is false, put an F in the space provided. If the answer is false, write in the correct answer to make it true.

15. _____ A warm-down consists of a slow jog or walk with some stretching.

16. _____ Your body as a teenager is indestructible.

17. _____ A warm-up or warm-down will help prevent injuries.

18. _____ The warm-up should last anywhere between 8-15 minutes.

19. _____ The first step in a proper warm-up is thoroughly stretching you muscles.

20. _____ When injured the first thing to do is get heat on the injury.

SHORT ANSWER: Answer the following questions.

21. Explain what is meant by the term "lifetime sports." (3 points)
    Lifetime sports are:

22. List 3 examples of lifetime sports. (3 points; 1 point each)

    3 examples include:

23. Explain why the most important measurement of your fitness is cardiovascular fitness. (5 points)

24. What is the important role that exercise has in controlling one's weight? (5 points)

25. How might you include more activity in your lifestyle? (5 points)

26. What is the difference between aerobic and anaerobic exercise? Give one example of each kind of activity. (3 points)

ESSAY: Answer the following question using complete sentences.

27. Many teens compare themselves with others. Give examples (at least 5) of areas where teens compare themselves with others. Include what might be your hardest personal area of comparison with others. Explain how comparison can be dangerous. Give suggestions as to how teenagers can overcome this harmful pattern and explain what God thinks about comparison. (15 points) *Use back of this page to complete your essay.*

Total Health •• Chapter 4 • Test Key

Unit 1: Physical Health   100 points

DEFINE: Define the following terms as they are defined in the text. (14 points; 2 points each)

1. Anaerobic: *short bursts of activity without the use of much oxygen*

2. Fitness: *the ability of your mind and body to work together to their highest possible level*

3. Aerobic: *when your muscles demand more oxygen than normal during exercise*

4. Atrophy: *when a long period of time lapses between workouts and the muscles decrease in size and strength*

5. Cardiovascular fitness: *the condition of the heart*

6. Muscular fitness: *the condition of your muscles' strength and endurance*

7. Flexibility: *the ability to have a full range of motion with your body parts*

SHORT ANSWER: Answer the following questions.

8. Explain what is meant by the phrase, "accidental workout". Include in your answer any accidental workouts that your personal life includes already. (3 points)
    An accidental workout means to increase your activity level when you don't even know you are doing it. It is making exercise and movement a fun and enjoyable part of your daily life. E.g., riding horses, bike riding, skateboarding, jump rope, etc.

9. List 6 benefits of exercise. (12 points; 2 points each)
    a. *increases strength, stamina*   d. *relieves depression*

    b. *reduces stress, tension*   e. *reduces body fat*

    c. *improves mental alertness*   f. *increases BMR*

    (more answers on page 80 in student text)

10. List 5 reasons why your joint muscle flexibility is important. (5 points; 1 point each)
    a. *reduces chance of injury*   d. *helps clear the mind*

    b. *helps coordination*   e. *improves circulation*

    c. *increases range of motion*   f. *makes you feel better, reduces tension; makes work easier*

11. List each step in the treatment of injuries following the acronym R.I.C.E. (4 points; 1 point each)

    Rest *the injured area.*

    Ice *the injured area to prevent swelling.*

    Compress *the injured area with a towel or bandage to prevent swelling.*

    Elevate *the injured area above the level of the heart to help drain fluid that might collect at the injury.*

12. Explain what is meant by the term "body composition"? (3 points)

    Body composition is: *the relationship between your fat and lean (muscle) body weight.*

13. Give 2 benefits to increasing your lean muscle weight. (4 points; 2 points each)

    Two benefits of increasing my lean muscle weight are:

    a. *burns more calories while you are at rest*

    b. *decreases your body fat*

14. Explain why the phrase, "No pain, No gain" is incorrect when it comes to stretching and exercise? (4 points)

    Because when it comes to terms of stretching and exercising, when your body feels pain, you are pushing it too far and toward potential injury. See example of Susan pushing herself too hard when in junior high on pages 91-92.

TRUE OR FALSE: (12 points; 2 points each) If the answer is true, put a T in the space provided. If the answer is false, put an F in the space provided. If the answer is false, write in the correct answer to make it true.

15. __T__ A warm-down consists of a slow jog or walk with some stretching.

16. __F__ Your body as a teenager is indestructible.

    No way! You can get hurt.

17. __T__ A warm-up or warm-down will help prevent injuries.

18. __T__ The warm-up should last anywhere between 8-15 minutes.

19. __F__ The first step in a proper warm-up is thoroughly stretching you muscles.

    light movement, large muscle groups

20. __F__ When injured the first thing to do is get heat on the injury.

    Ice

SHORT ANSWER: Answer the following questions.

21. Explain what is meant by the term "lifetime sports." (3 points)

    Lifetime sports are: *activities that a person can participate in throughout a lifetime*

22. List 3 examples of lifetime sports. (3 points; 1 point each)

    3 examples include: *tennis, walking, golf, jogging*

23. Explain why the most important measurement of your fitness is cardiovascular fitness. (5 points)

    A strong heart, along with healthy lungs and blood vessels work together to supply oxygenated blood to the whole body. Without good cardiovascular fitness, it would not matter how much weight you could lift if you died from a heart attack!

24. What is the important role that exercise has in controlling one's weight? (5 points)

    Exercise is very important when it comes to controlling weight because if you consume more calories than you burn, you will gain weight. Eating fatty foods and living a sedentary lifestyle will cause you to gain weight. But, you may actually gain weight as you exercise if you are losing fat and increasing your lean muscle mass.

25. How might you include more activity in your lifestyle? (5 points)

    Answers will vary. Look for them to record doable exercise(s) and/or activities that require movement and how they plan—or could plan—to incorporate them into their daily lifestyles.

26. What is the difference between aerobic and anaerobic exercise? Give one example of each kind of activity. (3 points)

    Aerobic exercise is when your body requires more oxygen than normal to do the activity, example, jogging. Anaerobic exercise consists of short bursts of energy without much use of oxygen by the body to accomplish the activity, example: weight lifting.

ESSAY: Answer the following question using complete sentences.

27. Many teens compare themselves with others. Give examples (at least 5) of areas where teens compare themselves with others. Include what might be your hardest personal area of comparison with others. Explain how comparison can be dangerous. Give suggestions as to how teenagers can overcome this harmful pattern and explain what God thinks about comparison. (15 points) *Use back of this page to complete your essay.*

    Answers will vary but could include the following: Teens compare in the areas of appearance (clothing, weight, hairstyles), intelligence (grades), money, popularity, athletic ability, music ability, and family life. Comparing is one of the greatest enemies to your mind because it will either make you feel superior to others who aren't as good as you, or make you feel inferior to others who are better than you. Teens can overcome this by thanking God for everything in their lives, reading the Word on God's unconditional love for them, asking God in prayer for help to overcome this attitude. God never intended for anybody to compare themselves with others. God only expects everyone to do their best and become the finest person they can become with the resources He's given to them.

Total Health • **Chapter 5 • Quiz A**

Unit 1: Physical Health   Name:_____

Sections 5.1-5.2   Date: _____

20 Points   Score: _____

MATCHING: (10 points; 1 point each) For each numbered item, place the letter of the correct answer in the space provided at the left of each item. Each answer can be used only once.

1. _____ Infectious disease
2. _____ Pathogens
3. _____ Virus
4. _____ Vaccine
5. _____ Bacteria
6. _____ Symptoms
7. _____ Antibodies
8. _____ Non-infectious disease
9. _____ Resident bacteria
10. _____ Lymphocytes

A. Stuffy nose, sore throat.
B. Germs.
C. White blood cells that fight off germs.
D. Friendly bacteria.
E. Diseases caused by heredity, environment, and/or lifestyle.
F. Produced by your white blood cells to fight off germs.
G. Diseases caused by germs that spread from one person to another.
H. Weakened or destroyed cells of a particular germ that is injected into a person to keep a person from getting the disease.
I. Single-celled organisms responsible for strep throat.
J. Small organisms responsible for the common cold, chicken pox and measles.

SHORT ANSWER: Answer the following questions.

11. List four ways that germs are spread. (4 points)
    a.
    b.
    c.
    d.

12. Explain why good bacteria are important for your body. (1 point)

13. How can you replace the good bacteria in your body? (1 point)

14. What is meant by the phrase "Listen to your body"? (2 points)

15. How are most germs carried and passed on to another human being? (1 point)

16. What can a person do to help decrease the spread of germs? (1 point)

Total Health · Chapter 5 • Quiz A Key

Unit 1: Physical Health

20 points

Sections 5.1-5.2

MATCHING: (10 points; 1 point each) For each numbered item, place the letter of the correct answer in the space provided at the left of each item. Each answer can be used only once.

1. _G_ Infectious disease
2. _B_ Pathogens
3. _J_ Virus
4. _H_ Vaccine
5. _I_ Bacteria
6. _A_ Symptoms
7. _F_ Antibodies
8. _E_ Non-infectious disease
9. _D_ Resident bacteria
10. _C_ Lymphocytes

A. Stuffy nose, sore throat.
B. Germs.
C. White blood cells that fight off germs.
D. Friendly bacteria.
E. Diseases caused by heredity, environment, and/or lifestyle.
F. Produced by your white blood cells to fight off germs.
G. Diseases caused by germs that spread from one person to another.
H. Weakened or destroyed cells of a particular germ that is injected into a person to keep a person from getting the disease.
I. Single-celled organisms responsible for strep throat.
J. Small organisms responsible for the common cold, chicken pox and measles.

SHORT ANSWER: Answer the following questions.

11. List four ways that germs are spread. (4 points)
    a. *contact with airborne germ*
    b. *contact with objects that an infected person has touched*
    c. *contact with an infected animal*
    d. *contact with an infected person*

12. Explain why good bacteria are important for your body. (1 point)
    Good or "friendly" bacteria grow in your intestines and are vital for proper digestion and strengthen your immune system.

13. How can you replace the good bacteria in your body? (1 point)
    Take "friendly flora" supplements as well as lots of yogurt that contains good bacteria.

14. What is meant by the phrase "Listen to your body"? (2 points)
    When you experience certain symptoms, or signals from your body that it might be fighting a bug, make sure you treat your body with plenty of water, rest and nutritious food.

15. How are most germs carried and passed on to another human being? (1 point)
    By way of the hands, touching things that have been handled by an infected person.

16. What can a person do to help decrease the spread of germs? (1 point)
    Wash your hands often!

Total Health ·································· Chapter 5 • Quiz B

Unit 1: Physical Health

Sections 5.3-5.4

25 Points

Name:_____

Date: _____

Score: _____

MATCHING: (10 points; 1 point each) For each numbered item, place the letter of the correct answer in the space provided at the left of each item. Each answer can be used only once.

1. _____ Tumor
2. _____ Congenital
3. _____ HIV
4. _____ STD
5. _____ Carcinogen
6. _____ Diabetes Type I
7. _____ Cancer
8. _____ AIDS
9. _____ Hypoglycemia
10. _____ Diabetes Type II

A. Sexually transmitted disease.
B. A disease which occurs when abnormal cells grow out of control.
C. A mass of abnormal cells.
D. A condition in which the pancreas releases too much insulin.
E. The virus that causes AIDS.
F. Non-insulin dependent diabetes.
G. Any substance that tends to produce cancer.
H. Insulin-dependent diabetes.
I. Occurring at birth.
J. Acquired Immunodeficiency Syndrome.

SHORT ANSWER AND FILL IN THE BLANK: Answer the following questions.

11. A person's strong belief on a particular issue is called a _____. (1 point)

12. _____ is a hormone produced by the pancreas to control how the body uses sugar. (1 point)

13. List 4 of the 5 factors that increase your chance of developing cancer. (4 points)

14. What is the only way to prevent getting a sexually transmitted disease? (1 point)

15. Explain why it is important to develop strong convictions about your personal sexual boundaries before you find yourself in a relationship with the opposite sex. (2 points)

16. List 4 of the 8 risk factors contributing to heart disease. (4 points)

17. What are 2 things that you can you do at a young age to prevent heart disease? (2 points)

Total Health •••••••••••••••••••••••••••••••••• Chapter 5 • Quiz B Key

Unit 1: Physical Health

25 points

Sections 5.3-5.4

MATCHING: (10 points; 1 point each) For each numbered item, place the letter of the correct answer in the space provided at the left of each item. Each answer can be used only once.

1. _C_ Tumor
2. _I_ Congenital
3. _E_ HIV
4. _A_ STD
5. _G_ Carcinogen
6. _H_ Diabetes Type I
7. _B_ Cancer
8. _J_ AIDS
9. _D_ Hypoglycemia
10. _F_ Diabetes Type II

A. Sexually transmitted disease.
B. A disease which occurs when abnormal cells grow out of control.
C. A mass of abnormal cells.
D. A condition in which the pancreas releases too much insulin.
E. The virus that causes AIDS.
F. Non-insulin dependent diabetes.
G. Any substance that tends to produce cancer.
H. Insulin-dependent diabetes.
I. Occurring at birth.
J. Acquired Immunodeficiency Syndrome.

SHORT ANSWER AND FILL IN THE BLANK: Answer the following questions.

11. A person's strong belief on a particular issue is called a ____conviction____. (1 point)

12. ____Insulin____ is a hormone produced by the pancreas to control how the body uses sugar. (1 point)

13. List 4 of the 5 factors that increase your chance of developing cancer. (4 points)
    a. *Genetic make-up (heredity)*
    b. *Lifestyle*
    c. *Occupational hazards*
    d. *Environmental factors*
    e. *The body's reaction to a virus*

14. What is the only way to prevent getting a sexually transmitted disease? (1 point)
    sexual abstinence

15. Explain why it is important to develop strong convictions about your personal sexual boundaries before you find yourself in a relationship with the opposite sex. (2 points)
    It is important to know what you believe and why you believe it before you find yourself in a compromising situation. Often people do things they will regret because they have not developed a strong conviction about it before the temptation faces them.

16. List 4 of the 8 risk factors contributing to heart disease. (4 points)
    a. *High blood pressure*
    b. *Smoking*
    c. *Obesity*
    d. *Stress*
    e. *High cholesterol*
    f. *Diabetes*
    g. *Lack of exercise*
    h. *Alcohol*

17. What are 2 things that you can you do at a young age to prevent heart disease? (2 points)
    a. *Discover your family's health history concerning heart disease.*
    b. *Have a healthy lifestyle that includes fresh fruits, vegetables; limit fats and salt.*
    c. *Exercise regularly.*
    d. *Decrease stress.*

Total Health • **Chapter 5 • Test**

Unit 1: Physical Health

100 Points

Name:_____

Date: _____

Score: _____

MATCHING: (20 points; 2 point each) For each numbered item, place the letter of the correct answer in the space provided at the left of each item. Each answer can be used only once.

1. _____ Infectious disease
2. _____ Pathogens
3. _____ Virus
4. _____ Vaccine
5. _____ Bacteria
6. _____ Symptoms
7. _____ Antibodies
8. _____ Non-infectious disease
9. _____ Resident bacteria
10. _____ Lymphocytes

A. Diseases caused by heredity, environment and/or lifestyle.

B. Diseases caused by germs that spread from one person to another.

C. White blood cells that fight off germs.

D. Germs.

E. Small organisms responsible for the common cold, chicken pox and measles.

F. Produced by your white blood cells to fight off germs.

G. Weakened or destroyed cells of a particular germ that is injected into a person to keep a person from getting the disease.

H. Friendly bacteria.

I. Stuffy nose, sore throat.

J. Single-celled organisms responsible for strep throat.

K. A group or mass of abnormal cells.

SHORT ANSWER: Answer the following questions.

11. How can you replace the good bacteria in your body? (3 points)

12. What is meant by the phrase "Listen to your body"? (3 points)

13. List 4 of the 8 risk factors contributing to heart disease. (8 points; 2 points each)

    a.   c.

    b.   d.

14. Explain why good bacteria are important for your body. (3 points)

MATCHING (20 points; 2 points each): For each numbered item, place the letter of the correct answer in the space provided at the left of each item. Each answer can be used only once.

15. _____ Tumor

16. _____ Congenital

17. _____ HIV

18. _____ STD

19. _____ Carcinogen

20. _____ Diabetes Type I

21. _____ Cancer

22. _____ AIDS

23. _____ Hypoglycemia

24. _____ Diabetes Type II

A. Insulin-dependent diabetes.

B. Acquired Immunodeficiency Syndrome.

C. Masses of abnormal cells.

D. Sexually transmitted disease.

E. Non-insulin dependent diabetes.

F. A disease which occurs when abnormal cells grow out of control.

G. A condition in which the pancreas releases too much insulin.

H. The virus that causes AIDS.

I. Any substance that tends to produce cancer.

J. Occurring at birth.

K. The need for internal balance.

SHORT ANSWER OR FILL IN THE BLANK

25. A person's strong belief on a particular issue is called a _____. (3 points)

26. How are most germs carried and passed on to another human being? (3 points)

27. List 4 of the 5 factors that increase your chance of developing cancer. (4 points)

    a.

    b.

    c.

    d.

28. What is the only way to prevent getting a sexually transmitted disease? (2 point)

29. What can a person do to help decrease the spread of germs? (1 point)

30. _____ is a hormone produced by the pancreas to control how the body uses sugar. (1 point)

31. Explain why it is important to develop strong convictions about your personal sexual boundaries before you find yourself in a relationship with the opposite sex. (4 points)

32. What can you learn from Kristen's (the teen who died from bone cancer at 15 years of age) attitude about life? (5 points)

33. How might Kristen's story relate to James 1:17, "Every good gift and every prefect gift is from above and comes down from the Father of lights..."? (5 points)

34. What other (spiritual) defenses do you have as a Christian to fight off disease and sickness? (3 points)

ESSAY: Answer the following question using full sentences.

35. As you evaluate your present lifestyle, what aspects could you change to help to prevent disease as you get older? (12 points) *Use back of this page to complete your essay.*

Total Health · Chapter 5 • Test Key

Unit 1: Physical Health   100 points

MATCHING: (20 points; 2 point each) For each numbered item, place the letter of the correct answer in the space provided at the left of each item. Each answer can be used only once.

1. _B_ Infectious disease
2. _D_ Pathogens
3. _E_ Virus
4. _G_ Vaccine
5. _J_ Bacteria
6. _I_ Symptoms
7. _F_ Antibodies
8. _A_ Non-infectious disease
9. _H_ Resident bacteria
10. _C_ Lymphocytes

A. Diseases caused by heredity, environment and/or lifestyle.
B. Diseases caused by germs that spread from one person to another.
C. White blood cells that fight off germs.
D. Germs.
E. Small organisms responsible for the common cold, chicken pox and measles.
F. Produced by your white blood cells to fight off germs.
G. Weakened or destroyed cells of a particular germ that is injected into a person to keep a person from getting the disease.
H. Friendly bacteria.
I. Stuffy nose, sore throat.
J. Single-celled organisms responsible for strep throat.
K. A group or mass of abnormal cells.

SHORT ANSWER: Answer the following questions.

11. How can you replace the good bacteria in your body? (3 points)
Take "friendly flora" supplements as well as lots of yogurt that contains good bacteria.

12. What is meant by the phrase "Listen to your body"? (3 points)
When you experience certain symptoms, or signals from your body that it might be fighting a bug, make sure you treat your body with plenty of water, rest and nutritious food.

13. List 4 of the 8 risk factors contributing to heart disease. (8 points; 2 points each)
a. *High blood pressure*   c. *Obesity*
b. *Smoking*   d. *Stress*
high cholesterol, diabetes, lack of exercise, alcohol

14. Explain why good bacteria are important for your body. (3 points)
Good or "friendly" bacteria grow in your intestines and are vital for proper digestion and strengthen your immune system.

MATCHING (20 points; 2 points each): For each numbered item, place the letter of the correct answer in the space provided at the left of each item. Each answer can be used only once.

15. _C_ Tumor
16. _J_ Congenital
17. _H_ HIV
18. _D_ STD
19. _I_ Carcinogen
20. _A_ Diabetes Type I
21. _F_ Cancer
22. _B_ AIDS
23. _G_ Hypoglycemia
24. _E_ Diabetes Type II

A. Insulin-dependent diabetes.
B. Acquired Immunodeficiency Syndrome.
C. Masses of abnormal cells.
D. Sexually transmitted disease.
E. Non-insulin dependent diabetes.
F. A disease which occurs when abnormal cells grow out of control.
G. A condition in which the pancreas releases too much insulin.
H. The virus that causes AIDS.
I. Any substance that tends to produce cancer.
J. Occurring at birth.
K. The need for internal balance.

SHORT ANSWER OR FILL IN THE BLANK

25. A person's strong belief on a particular issue is called a ___conviction___. (3 points)

26. How are most germs carried and passed on to another human being? (3 points)
    By way of the hands, touching things that have been handled by an infected person.

27. List 4 of the 5 factors that increase your chance of developing cancer. (4 points)
    a. *Genetic make-up (heredity)*
    b. *Lifestyle*
    c. *Occupational hazards*
    d. *Environmental factors*
    The body's reaction to a virus

28. What is the only way to prevent getting a sexually transmitted disease? (2 point)
    sexual abstinence

29. What can a person do to help decrease the spread of germs? (1 point)
    Wash your hands often!

30. ___Insulin___ is a hormone produced by the pancreas to control how the body uses sugar. (1 point)

31. Explain why it is important to develop strong convictions about your personal sexual boundaries before you find yourself in a relationship with the opposite sex. (4 points)
    It is important to know what you believe and why you believe it before you find yourself in a compromising situation. Often people do things they will regret because they have not developed a strong conviction about it before the temptation faces them.

32. What can you learn from Kristen's (the teen who died from bone cancer at 15 years of age) attitude about life? (5 points)

    You can learn that most of us take our good health for granted; that none of us know what is going to happen to us tomorrow.

33. How might Kristen's story relate to James 1:17, "Every good gift and every prefect gift is from above and comes down from the Father of lights..."? (5 points)

    All of our lives are good gifts from God. We need to appreciate what we have for as long as we have it and live with a grateful heart unto God as our creator, father, and source.

34. What other (spiritual) defenses do you have as a Christian to fight off disease and sickness? (3 points)

    Christians have God's Word which tells them what is healthy behavior and what it not, , faith in God's healing power, and faith in God's sovereign control.

ESSAY: Answer the following question using full sentences.

35. As you evaluate your present lifestyle, what aspects could you change to help to prevent disease as you get older? (12 points) *Use back of this page to complete your essay.*

    Discover whether there's heart disease, etc. in you family health history, get regular exercise, eat a nutritious diet (stay away from high fat, high salt, and high sugar foods), don't smoke, don't drink alcohol, stay at your ideal weight, learn to manage the stress in your life.

Total Health ••••••••••••••••••••••••••••••••••••••• Chapter 6 • Quiz A

Unit 2: Mental Health

Sections 6.1-6.2

20 Points

Name:_____

Date: _____

Score: _____

DEFINE: (5 points; 1 point each) Define the following terms as they are defined in the text.

1. Confident:

2. Personal identity:

3. Jealousy:

4. Mature:

5. Pride:

6. List one change you may be experiencing for each area in your life. (4 points)
    a. Physical:

    b. Mental (emotional):

    c. Social:

    d. Spiritual:

7. Explain how you can begin to replace feelings of worry with feelings of faith and trust in God. (2 points)

8. Explain why God warns us against comparison and jealousy. (4 points)

9. Imagine that a friend of yours comes to you and asks, "If God really loves me, why did He let my parents split up?" What would you say to him or her? (5 points)

Total Health ························· Chapter 6 • Quiz A Key

Unit 2: Mental Health   20 points

Sections 6.1-6.2

DEFINE: (5 points; 1 point each) Define the following terms as they are defined in the text.

1. Confident: *no feelings of inferiority*

2. Personal identity: *to know who you are in Christ*

3. Jealousy: *feelings of resentment against another for having a success or talent that you want to have*

4. Mature: *grow physically, mentally, emotionally, socially, and spiritually*

5. Pride: *to think of yourself better than you really are; an "I don't need anyone" attitude*

6. List one change you may be experiencing for each area in your life. (4 points)

    a. Physical: *possible acne, increase in height and weight, needing to shower more often*

    b. Mental (emotional): *increased stress, feelings of independence, inability to "relate" to adults and that general feeling that "no one understands"*

    c. Social: *possible increase of tension at home, attraction to the opposite sex, increased peer pressure, and the desire for more freedom*

    d. Spiritual: *an overall sense of "I want to get closer to God but I don't know how", or other questions about God's role in your life*

7. Explain how you can begin to replace feelings of worry with feelings of faith and trust in God. (2 points)

    First, identify your worries, starting with the greatest one. After you realize what the greatest source of worry is right now, share it with God. As you are talking with God, take the time just to listen to what He says to you in your mind and in your heart. He will give you a sense of peace about your concern. Next, talk to someone you can trust, preferably an adult.

8. Explain why God warns us against comparison and jealousy. (4 points)

    Comparison and jealousy ruin relationships. They put a big wedge between you and the other person. They also affect your thoughts about yourself. Possibly worst of all, they can lead you into pride—thinking that you are better than others. If you have a problem with jealousy, talk to God about the way you feel. Ask Him to help you to overcome comparison and be grateful for all that He has done for you.

9. Imagine that a friend of yours comes to you and asks, "If God really loves me, why did He let my parents split up?" What would you say to him or her? (5 points)

    Sometimes bad things happen to Christians just like non-Christians. Many times you don't understand why things happen. There is no easy answer for this, but God has a unique way of causing good to come from bad. I know it is hard right now, but if you turn to God and share your true feelings with Him, He will help you through this time.

Total Health · Chapter 6 • Quiz B

Unit 2: Mental Health

Section 6.3

20 Points

Name:_____

Date: _____

Score: _____

DEFINE: (4 points; 2 points each) Define the following terms as they are defined in the text.

1. What is character?

2. What is self-esteem?

SHORT ANSWER: (12 points; 3 points each) Respond to the following teen quotes using principles you have learned. Try to apply a Bible character in the text to each answer.

3. "I feel that I'm mature enough to handle more responsibility. Why aren't my parents letting me have more privileges?"

4. "I don't have anyone to talk to. Nobody understands me. I want to handle things on my own."

5. "Sometimes I get angry about the things my brother does to me. What should I do?"

6. "I really want to be friends with the popular kids in my class. Sometimes they are really nice to me and other times they are so mean. I find I can't be myself around them. Why do I want to be their friend, anyway, since they are so mean to me?"

SHORT ANSWER: (4 points):

7. Explain the following diagram.

Total isolation ——————————————→ secrecy

Secrecy ——————————————→ deception

Deception ——————————————→ sin

Sin ——————————————→ self-destruction

Total Health · **Chapter 6 • Quiz B Key**

Unit 2: Mental Health   20 points

Section 6.3

DEFINE: (4 points; 2 points each) Define the following terms as they are defined in the text.

1. What is character? *What you are on the inside; what you do when no one is watching*

2. What is self-esteem? *The way you feel about yourself*

SHORT ANSWER: (12 points; 3 points each) Respond to the following teen quotes using principles you have learned. Try to apply a Bible character in the text to each answer.

Answers may vary but the general theme for each illustration may include:

3. "I feel that I'm mature enough to handle more responsibility. Why aren't my parents letting me have more privileges?"

    The Faithful Servant theme: faithfulness in present responsibilities leads to an increase in your personal responsibilities. He who is faithful in little, will be faithful in much.

4. "I don't have anyone to talk to. Nobody understands me. I want to handle things on my own."

    Judas: Avoid secrecy and isolation.

    King David: Grow in openness to God.

5. "Sometimes I get angry about the things my brother does to me. What should I do?"

    Joseph: Learn how to forgive those who hurt you.

6. "I really want to be friends with the popular kids in my class. Sometimes they are really nice to me and other times they are so mean. I find I can't be myself around them. Why do I want to be their friend, anyway, since they are so mean to me?"

    Samuel: Focus on what really matters. Man looks on the outward, but God looks at the heart.

    Peter: Grow in your possession of stand-alone courage.

SHORT ANSWER: (4 points):

7. Explain the following diagram.

Total isolation ⟶ secrecy
Secrecy ⟶ deception
Deception ⟶ sin
Sin ⟶ self-destruction

If you allow yourself to become isolated from the positive influence of other strong Christians, it will give Satan greater freedom to deceive you. Eventually, the result will be manifested in your actions—sin. While Satan wants to make you believe that you can and should handle all of your problems and temptations on your own, that's not the way God made you. God made you to need other Christians for strength, encouragement, counsel, and prayer.

Total Health · Chapter 6 • Test

Unit 2: Mental Health

Name:_____

100 Points

Date: _____

Score: _____

DEFINE: (21 points; 3 points each) Define the following terms as they are defined in the text.

1. Mature:

2. Jealousy:

3. Character:

4. Self-esteem:

5. Confident:

6. Pride:

7. Personal identity:

SHORT ANSWER: Answer the following questions.

8. Imagine that a friend of yours comes to you and asks, "If God really loves me, then why did He let my parents split up?" What would you say to him or her? (5 points)

Respond to the following teen quotes (questions 9-12) using principles you have learned.

9. "I don't have anyone to talk to. Nobody understands me. I want to handle things on my own." (5 points)

10. "I feel that I'm mature enough to handle more responsibility. Why aren't my parents letting me have more privileges?" (5 points)

11. "Sometimes I get angry about the things my brother does to me. What should I do?" (5 points)

12. "I really want to be friends with the popular kids in my class. Sometimes they are really nice to me and other times they are so mean. I find I can't be myself around them. Why do I want to be their friend, anyway, since they are so mean to me?" (5 points)

13. List one change you may be experiencing for each area in your life. (8 points; 2 points each)
    a. Physical:

    b. Mental (emotional):

    c. Social:

    d. Spiritual:

14. Explain the following diagram. (8 points; 2 points for each line):

    Total isolation ⟶ secrecy
    Secrecy ⟶ deception
    Deception ⟶ sin
    Sin ⟶ self-destruction

15. Choose *three* of the following biblical illustrations and, according to the text, explain what principle(s) of life can be learned from their example: (15 points; 5 points each)

   A. The Faithful Servant (Luke 16:10):

   B. Samuel (I Samuel 16:7):

   C. King David (Psalm 22:1; 124:7):

   D. Judas (Matthew 26:14-16):

   E. Joseph (Genesis 37:4, 39:20; 40:23):

   F. Peter (Mark 14:66-72; Acts 3:11-26):

16. List the four main reasons that the text gives—in the section, "Why All These Changes?"—for why the Lord is now allowing so many different changes to come into your life. (5 points)
   a.

   b.

   c.

   d.

17. Explain why God warns us against jealousy. Include in your answer your own experiences with jealousy, examples of where teens may be jealous of others, and how a teen can overcome jealousy. (8 points)

ESSAY: Answer the following question(s) using complete sentences.

18. Explain how you can begin to replace feelings of worry with feelings of faith and trust in God. (10 points)

EXTRA CREDIT

Read Jeremiah 18:3-4 about the potter and the clay. Describe the process required to create a beautiful vessel. Apply this truth to the changes taking place in your own life. (5 points)

Total Health • **Chapter 6 • Test Key**

Unit 2: Mental Health   100 points

DEFINE: (21 points; 3 points each) Define the following terms as they are defined in the text.

1. Mature: *grow physically, mentally, emotionally, socially, and spiritually*

2. Jealousy: *feeling of resentment against another for having a success or talent that you want to have*

3. Character: *What you are on the inside; what you do when no one is watching*

4. Self-esteem: *The way you feel about yourself*

5. Confident: *no feelings of inferiority*

6. Pride: *to think of yourself better than you really are; an "I don't need anyone" attitude*

7. Personal identity: *to know who you are in Christ*

SHORT ANSWER: Answer the following questions.

8. Imagine that a friend of yours comes to you and asks, "If God really loves me, then why did He let my parents split up?" What would you say to him or her? (5 points)

   Sometimes bad things happen to Christians just like non-Christians. Many times you don't understand why things happen. There is no easy answer for this, but God has a unique way of causing good to come from bad. I know it is hard right now, but if you turn to God and share your true feelings with Him, He will help you through this time.

Respond to the following teen quotes (questions 9-12) using principles you have learned.

Answers may vary but the general theme for each illustration may the biblical illustrations from the text:

9. "I don't have anyone to talk to. Nobody understands me. I want to handle things on my own." (5 points)

   Judas: Avoid secrecy and isolation.

   King David: Grow in openness to God.

10. "I feel that I'm mature enough to handle more responsibility. Why aren't my parents letting me have more privileges?" (5 points)

    The Faithful Servant theme: faithfulness in present responsibilities leads to an increase in your personal responsibilities. He who is faithful in little, will be faithful in much.

11. "Sometimes I get angry about the things my brother does to me. What should I do?" (5 points)

    Joseph: Learn how to forgive those who hurt you.

12. "I really want to be friends with the popular kids in my class. Sometimes they are really nice to me and other times they are so mean. I find I can't be myself around them. Why do I want to be their friend, anyway, since they are so mean to me?" (5 points)

    Samuel: Focus on what really matters. Man looks on the outward, but God looks at the heart.
    Peter: Grow in your possession of stand-alone courage.

13. List one change you may be experiencing for each area in your life. (8 points; 2 points each)

    a. Physical: *possible acne, increase in height and weight, needing to shower more often*

    b. Mental (emotional): *increased stress, feelings of independence, inability to "relate" to adults and that general feeling that "no one understands"*

    c. Social: *possible increase of tension at home, attraction to the opposite sex, increased peer pressure, and the desire for more freedom*

    d. Spiritual: *an overall sense of "I want to get closer to God but I don't know how", or other questions about God's role in your own life.*

14. Explain the following diagram. (8 points; 2 points for each line):

    Total isolation ————————→ secrecy
    Secrecy ————————→ deception
    Deception ————————→ sin
    Sin ————————→ self-destruction

    If you allow yourself to become isolated from the positive influence of other strong Christians, it will give Satan greater freedom to deceive you. Eventually, the result will be manifested in your actions—sin. While Satan wants to make you believe that you can and should handle all of your problems and temptations on your own, that's not the way God made you. God made you to need other Christians for strength, encouragement, counsel, and prayer.

98

15. Choose *three* of the following biblical illustrations and, according to the text, explain what principle(s) of life can be learned from their example: (15 points; 5 points each)

    A. The Faithful Servant (Luke 16:10): *Faithfulness in fulfilling smaller responsibilities leads to gaining larger privileges.*

    B. Samuel (I Samuel 16:7): *We need to focus on what really matters. God doesn't look on the outward appearance. He looks on the heart.*

    C. King David (Psalm 22:1; 124:7): *We can get closer to God if we are open and honest with Him concerning our feelings.*

    D. Judas (Matthew 26:14-16): *Isolation and secrecy spell danger.*

    E. Joseph (Genesis 37:4, 39:20; 40:23): *We can learn to forgive those who have hurt and/or offended us. God brings good out of evil.*

    F. Peter (Mark 14:66-72; Acts 3:11-26): *God can take the cowardly and turn them into those with stand-alone courage.*

16. List the four main reasons that the text gives—in the section, "Why All These Changes?"—for why the Lord is now allowing so many different changes to come into your life. (5 points)

    a. *to become more like Christ*

    b. *to develop personal identity*

    c. *to develop confidence*

    d. *to develop openness*

17. Explain why God warns us against jealousy. Include in your answer your own experiences with jealousy, examples of where teens may be jealous of others, and how a teen can overcome jealousy. (8 points)

    Comparison and jealousy ruin relationships. They put a big wedge between you and the other person. They also affect your thoughts about yourself. Possibly worst of all, they can lead you into pride—thinking that you are better than others are. If you have a problem with jealousy, talk to God about the way you feel. Ask Him to help you to overcome comparison and be grateful for all that He has done for you.

99

ESSAY: Answer the following question(s) using complete sentences.

18. Explain how you can begin to replace feelings of worry with feelings of faith and trust in God. (10 points)

   First, identify your worries, starting with the greatest one. After you realize what the greatest source of worry is right now, share it with God. As you are talking with God, take the time just to listen to what He says to you in your mind and in your heart. He will give you a sense of peace about your concern. Next, talk to someone you can trust, preferably an adult.

EXTRA CREDIT

Read Jeremiah 18:3-4 about the potter and the clay. Describe the process required to create a beautiful vessel. Apply this truth to the changes taking place in your own life. (5 points)

   Life applications will vary. The potter decides on the purpose for the vessel; he molds it into the shape that he wants; he puts it into the fire; he may put it into the fire many times; he places it in a dark room to "set"; he brings it out into the light and it begins to fulfill its purpose.

Total Health · Chapter 7 • Quiz A

Unit 2: Mental Health

Sections 7.1-7.2 (through p. 155)

25 Points

Name:_____

Date: _____

Score: _____

MATCHING: (6 points; 1 point each) For each numbered item, place the letter of the correct answer in the space provided at the left of each item. Each answer can be used only once.

1. _____ Boundary

2. _____ Long-term goal

3. _____ Distract

4. _____ Short-term goal

5. _____ Self-control

6. _____ Goal(s)

A. To divide the mind.

B. An achievement toward which you work. Your personal aim, purpose, or end in doing or not doing something.

C. Something that you make specific plans to accomplish within a relatively brief period of time.

D. An invisible line that separates you from everyone and everything else; like a fence with a gate that you control between you and the outside world.

E. Something that you make specific plans to get done over a relatively long period of time.

F. Being able to restrain your words or behaviors that might hurt you or someone else.

SHORT ANSWER: Answer the following questions.

7. What are 2 ways that society defines success? (2 points)

8. What are 4 ways that God has given to you that can help you to make wise decisions? (4 points)

9. What is the easiest part about staying focused on a goal? (1 point)

10. What is the most difficult part of staying focused on a goal? (1 point)

11. List 4 practical ways that can help you to stay mentally focused. (4 points)

12. Concerning Chad's advice about the need of having self-control when he climbs:
    a. What did Chad say was his reason for not wanting to take a shortcut? (1 point)

    b. What do beginning climbers have a tendency of doing to escape their inner fears? (1 point)

13. What are boundaries? (1 point)

14. Why are they important in your life? (1 point)

15. What are two examples of a short-term goal? (1 point; $^1/_2$ point each)

16. What are two examples of a long-term goal? (1 point; $^1/_2$ point each)

17. What goals should you keep as Number One in your life? ($^1/_2$ point)

18. What did Christina say made her feel proud of herself when she achieved a goal? ($^1/_2$ point)

Total Health •••••••••••••••••••••••••••••••••• Chapter 7 • Quiz A Key

Unit 2: Mental Health   25 points

Sections 7.1-7.2 (through p. 155)

MATCHING: (6 points; 1 point each) For each numbered item, place the letter of the correct answer in the space provided at the left of each item. Each answer can be used only once.

1. __D__ Boundary
2. __E__ Long-term goal
3. __A__ Distract
4. __C__ Short-term goal
5. __F__ Self-control
6. __B__ Goal(s)

A. To divide the mind.

B. An achievement toward which you work. Your personal aim, purpose, or end in doing or not doing something.

C. Something that you make specific plans to accomplish within a relatively brief period of time.

D. An invisible line that separates you from everyone and everything else; like a fence with a gate that you control between you and the outside world.

E. Something that you make specific plans to get done over a relatively long period of time.

F. Being able to restrain your words or behaviors that might hurt you or someone else.

SHORT ANSWER: Answer the following questions.

7. What are 2 ways that society defines success? (2 points)

   money, fame/popularity

8. What are 4 ways that God has given to you that can help you to make wise decisions? (4 points)

   Learn from other's experiences, get input from mature adults you trust, take time to think about your decisions, pray for wisdom.

9. What is the easiest part about staying focused on a goal? (1 point)

   The easiest part is…staying focused on those activities you enjoy.

10. What is the most difficult part of staying focused on a goal? (1 point)

    The most difficult part is…staying focused on those activities you don't really enjoy but know you would be more successful if you did, e.g., homework.

11. List 4 practical ways that can help you to stay mentally focused. (4 points)

    wear earplugs while studying, reward yourself for completing your homework, don't do home-work in front of the TV/VCR, study in a library instead of at home, begin using a student calendar with a place for assignments, set up a general daily schedule with a friend and stick to it for at least a week, don't talk on the phone until after you've done all your chores

12. Concerning Chad's advice about the need of having self-control when he climbs:

    a. What did Chad say was his reason for not wanting to take a shortcut? (1 point)

    "I'll leave my route and get stuck."

    b. What do beginning climbers have a tendency of doing to escape their inner fears? (1 point)

    To climb just as fast as they can.

13. What are boundaries? (1 point)

    Boundaries are like gates between you and the outside world.

14. Why are they important in your life? (1 point)

    They are important because they: help you to prevent people from hurting you physically or emotionally; stop you from hurting others' feelings; give you a way of protecting yourself by being able to say, "No".

15. What are two examples of a short-term goal? (1 point; ½ point each)

    getting your homework done on time, calling your friend within two days, making every team practice this season, doing your daily chores.

16. What are two examples of a long-term goal? (1 point; ½ point each)

    planning on graduating from high school, looking forward to marriage after you get out of college, saving money to buy your first car

17. What goals should you keep as Number One in your life? (½ point)

    your spiritual goals

18. What did Christina say made her feel proud of herself when she achieved a goal? (½ point)

    doing the best that she could do at what she really wanted to do

Total Health • **Chapter 7 • Quiz B**

Unit 2: Mental Health

Sections 7.2 (from p. 155)-7.3

20 Points

Name:_____

Date: _____

Score: _____

SHORT ANSWER AND FILL IN THE BLANK: Answer the following questions.

1. Your present interest or hobby could be a key to your _____. (1 point)

2. The main goal that teachers want you to reach in school is a _____. (3 points)

3. What is the reason that it is good to love to learn? (1 point)

4. What are three things that lifelong learners do? (3 points)

5. Write out the New Testament verse which tells us that no matter how much we think we know, that we can always learn more. (1 point)

TRUE OR FALSE:

Place either a T for true or a F for false in front of each of the following statements according to the text's description of the concept of "motivation". (4 points; 1 point each)

6. _____ It is an inner urge or motor.

7. _____ It does not prompt you to do what others would be afraid to do.

8. _____ It sometimes comes directly from God.

9. _____ It's different from an outward "incentive" which promises you friends or money to get you to do something.

Place either a T for true or a F for false in front of each of the following statements according to the text's description of what you should check when you feel bored or unmotivated. (3 points; 1 point each)

10. _____ You should check your motives.

11. _____ You should check your friendships.

12. _____ You should check your sleeping habits.

MULTIPLE CHOICE: Place a check in the box next to the one, best answer to the following question:

13. What was the main good result that came to the nation of Israel after God sent them into the Babylonian Captivity for their continual sin? (1 point)
   ❑ As a nation, they never slid back into idolatry.
   ❑ They were able to bring out of Babylon wealth they used to rebuild the temple.
   ❑ They had the opportunity of copying and distributing the Ten Commandments to their children.
   ❑ As a nation, they developed a new form of writing they used in writing some of the Old Testament.

SHORT ANSWER: Answer the following questions.

14. How would you describe the difference between a sin and a mistake? (1 point)

15. When you sin, how do you think Satan wants you to feel? (1 point)

16. How does this differ from the way God wants you to feel? (1 point)

Total Health ·············· Chapter 7 • Quiz B Key

Unit 2: Mental Health   20 points

Sections 7.2 (from p. 155)-7.3

SHORT ANSWER AND FILL IN THE BLANK: Answer the following questions.

1. Your present interest or hobby could be a key to your ____*future success*____. (1 point)
2. The main goal that teachers want you to reach in school is a ____*love for learning*____. (3 points)
3. What is the reason that it is good to love to learn? (1 point)

   If students can begin to love to learn, then they can do well at whatever they attempt. They'll be self-motivated to learn whatever they need to learn in order to be a success. This will be true whether they're inside or outside of a classroom.

4. What are three things that lifelong learners do? (3 points)

   Lifelong learners: develop critical thinking skills (discernment); grow in their awareness about the future (God's will and plans for them); increase their research skills (information retrieval)

5. Write out the New Testament verse which tells us that no matter how much we think we know, that we can always learn more. (1 point)

   I Corinthians 8:2, "And if anyone thinks that he knows anything, he knows nothing yet as he ought to know."

TRUE OR FALSE:

Place either a T for true or a F for false in front of each of the following statements according to the text's description of the concept of "motivation". (4 points; 1 point each)

6. _T_ It is an inner urge or motor.
7. _F_ It does not prompt you to do what others would be afraid to do.
8. _T_ It sometimes comes directly from God.
9. _T_ It's different from an outward "incentive" which promises you friends or money to get you to do something.

Place either a T for true or a F for false in front of each of the following statements according to the text's description of what you should check when you feel bored or unmotivated. (3 points; 1 point each)

10. _T_ You should check your motives. (1 point)

11. _T_ You should check your friendships. (1 point)

12. _F_ You should check your sleeping habits. (1 point)

MULTIPLE CHOICE: Place a check in the box next to the one, best answer to the following question:

13. What was the main good result that came to the nation of Israel after God sent them into the Babylonian Captivity for their continual sin? (1 point)

☑ As a nation, they never slid back into idolatry.

❑ They were able to bring out of Babylon wealth they used to rebuild the temple.

❑ They had the opportunity of copying and distributing the Ten Commandments to their children.

❑ As a nation, they developed a new form of writing they used in writing some of the Old Testament.

SHORT ANSWER: Answer the following questions.

14. How would you describe the difference between a sin and a mistake? (1 point)

If you were to cheat on a math test it would be a sin, but if you got an answer wrong on your math test just because you forgot how to do the problem or did not understand, then it would be a mistake but not a sin. A sin is a moral or spiritual transgression, contradictory to God's nature and His laws. A mistake is not a sin.

15. When you sin, how do you think Satan wants you to feel? (1 point)

Satan wants you to feel depressed, fearful and unmotivated to change. This keeps you away from God and others. Satan wants to keep you away from God and others who might help you. Satan wants you to harden your heart.

16. How does this differ from the way God wants you to feel? (1 point)

God wants you to have a heart that is willing to change. God wants you to go to Him and others immediately and not to wait. He wants to help you learn from your mistakes and cause good to come from them.

Total Health ··············· Chapter 7 • Test

Unit 2: Mental Health

100 Points

Name:_____

Date: _____

Score: _____

MATCHING: (6 points; 1 point each) For each numbered item, place the letter of the correct answer in the space provided at the left of each item. Each answer can be used only once.

1. _____ Boundary

2. _____ Long-term goal

3. _____ Distract

4. _____ Short-term goal

5. _____ Self-control

6. _____ Goal(s)

A. Something that you make specific plans to accomplish within a relatively brief period of time.

B. To divide the mind.

C. Something that you make specific plans to accomplish within a relatively brief period of time.

D. An achievement toward which you work. Your personal aim, purpose, or end in doing or not doing something. between you and the outside world.

E. An invisible line that separates you from everyone and everything else; like a fence with a gate that you control.

F. Being able to restrain your words or behaviors that might hurt you or someone else.

SHORT ANSWER AND FILL IN THE BLANK

7. What are two ways that society defines success? (2 points; 1 point each)

8. Your present interest or hobby could be a key to your _____. (2 points)

9. What are four ways that God has given to you that can help you to make wise decisions? (8 points; 2 points each)

   a.   c.

   b.   d.

10. The main goal that teachers want you to reach in school is a love for learning. What is the reason that it is good to love to learn? (2 points)

11. When you sin, how do you think Satan wants you to feel? (3 points)

109

12. How does this differ from the way God wants you to feel? (3 points)

13. List four practical ways that can help you to stay mentally focused. (8 points; 2 points each)

    a.

    b.

    c.

    d.

14. Why are boundaries important in your life? (3 points)

15. How would you describe the difference between a sin and a mistake? (3 points)

16. What goals should you keep as Number One in your life? (3 points)

17. What are three things that lifelong learners do? (6 points; 2 points each)

    a.

    b.

    c.

18. What are two examples of a short-term goal? (4 points; 2 points each)

    a.

    b.

19. Write out the New Testament verse, which tells us that no matter how much we think we know that we can always learn more. (2 points)

20. What are two examples of a long-term goal? (4 points; 2 points each)

    a.

    b.

TRUE OR FALSE: Place either a T for true or an F for false in front of each of the following statements according to the text's description of the concept of "motivation". (8 points; 2 points each)

21. _____ Motivation is different from an outward "incentive" which promises you friends or money to get you to do something.

22. _____ Motivation sometimes comes directly from God.

23. _____ Motivation does not prompt you to do what others would be afraid to do.

24. _____ Motivation is an inner urge or motor.

Place either a T for true or a F for false in front of each of the following statements according to the text's description of what you should check when you feel bored or unmotivated. (6 points; 2 points each)

25. _____ You should check your sleeping habits.

26. _____ You should check your motives.

27. _____ You should check your friendships.

MULTIPLE CHOICE: Place a check in the box next to the one, best answer to the following question:

28. What was the main good result that came to the nation of Israel after God sent them into the Babylonian Captivity for their continual sin? (1 point)

    ❏ They had the opportunity of copying and distributing the Ten Commandments to their children.

    ❏ They were able to bring out of Babylon wealth they used to rebuild the temple.

    ❏ As a nation, they never slid back into idolatry.

    ❏ As a nation, they developed a new form of writing they used in writing some of the Old Testament.

SHORT ANSWER: Answer the following questions.

29. Name three areas of your life where you believe you could become more focused. (6 points; 2 points each)

    a.

    b.

    c.

30. Explain what personal changes you could make in each area you mentioned above to help you stay focused. (6 points; 2 points each)

    a.

    b.

    c.

ESSAY: Answer the following question using complete sentences.

31. How might you apply the seven steps to success from the text to your own personal life? Include in your answer each of the seven steps and one application to your life for each of the steps. (14 points; 2 points each)

    (1)

    (2)

    (3)

    (4)

    (5)

    (6)

    (7)

Total Health • Chapter 7 • Test Key

Unit 2: Mental Health   100 points

MATCHING: (6 points; 1 point each) For each numbered item, place the letter of the correct answer in the space provided at the left of each item. Each answer can be used only once.

1. __E__ Boundary
2. __A__ Long-term goal
3. __B__ Distract
4. __C__ Short-term goal
5. __F__ Self-control
6. __D__ Goal(s)

A. Something that you make specific plans to accomplish within a relatively brief period of time.

B. To divide the mind.

C. Something that you make specific plans to accomplish within a relatively brief period of time.

D. An achievement toward which you work. Your personal aim, purpose, or end in doing or not doing something. between you and the outside world.

E. An invisible line that separates you from everyone and everything else; like a fence with a gate that you control.

F. Being able to restrain your words or behaviors that might hurt you or someone else.

SHORT ANSWER AND FILL IN THE BLANK

7. What are two ways that society defines success? (2 points; 1 point each)

   money, fame/popularity

8. Your present interest or hobby could be a key to your ____*future success*____. (2 points)

9. What are four ways that God has given to you that can help you to make wise decisions? (8 points; 2 points each)

   a. *Learn from others' experiences.*   c. *Pray for wisdom.*

   b. *Get input from mature adults you trust.*   d. *Take time to think about your decisions,*

10. The main goal that teachers want you to reach in school is a love for learning. What is the reason that it is good to love to learn? (2 points)

    If students can begin to love to learn, then they can do well at whatever they attempt. They'll be self-motivated to learn whatever they need to learn in order to be a success. This will be true whether they're inside or outside of a classroom.

11. When you sin, how do you think Satan wants you to feel? (3 points)

    Satan wants you to feel depressed, fearful and unmotivated to change. This keeps you away from God and others. Satan wants to keep you away from God and others who might help you. Satan wants you to harden your heart.

12. How does this differ from the way God wants you to feel? (3 points)

    God wants you to have a heart that is willing to change. God wants you to go to Him and others immediately and not to wait. He wants to help you learn from your mistakes and cause good to come from them.

13. List four practical ways that can help you to stay mentally focused. (8 points; 2 points each)

    a. wear earplugs while studying

    b. reward yourself for completing your homework

    c. don't do homework in front of the TV/VCR

    d. study in a library instead of at home

    e. begin using a student calendar with a place for assignments

    f. set up a general daily schedule with a friend and stick to it for at least a week

    g. don't talk on the phone until after you've done all your chores

14. Why are boundaries important in your life? (3 points)

    They are important because they: help you to prevent people from hurting you physically or emotionally; stop you from hurting other's feelings; give you a way of protecting yourself by being able to say, "No".

15. How would you describe the difference between a sin and a mistake? (3 points)

    If you were to cheat on a math test it would be a sin, but if you got an answer wrong on your math test just because you forgot how to do the problem or did not understand, then it would be a mistake but not a sin. A sin is a moral or spiritual transgression, contradictory to God's nature and His laws. A mistake is not a sin.

16. What goals should you keep as Number One in your life? (3 points)

    Your spiritual goals.

17. What are three things that lifelong learners do? (6 points; 2 points each)

    a. develop critical thinking skills (discernment)

    b. grow in their awareness about the future (God's will and plans for them)

    c. increase their research skills (information retrieval)

18. What are two examples of a short-term goal? (4 points; 2 points each)

    a. getting your homework done on time

    b. calling your friend within two days

    c. making every team practice this season

    d. doing your daily chores.

19. Write out the New Testament verse, which tells us that no matter how much we think we know that we can always learn more. (2 points)

    I Corinthians 8:2, "And if anyone thinks that he knows anything, he knows nothing yet as he ought to know."

20. What are two examples of a long-term goal? (4 points; 2 points each)

    a. planning on graduating from high school

    b. looking forward to marriage after you get out of college

    c. saving money to buy your first car.

TRUE OR FALSE: Place either a T for true or an F for false in front of each of the following statements according to the text's description of the concept of "motivation". (8 points; 2 points each)

21. _T_ Motivation is different from an outward "incentive" which promises you friends or money to get you to do something.

22. _T_ Motivation sometimes comes directly from God.

23. _F_ Motivation does not prompt you to do what others would be afraid to do.

24. _T_ Motivation is an inner urge or motor.

Place either a T for true or a F for false in front of each of the following statements according to the text's description of what you should check when you feel bored or unmotivated. (6 points; 2 points each)

25. _F_ You should check your sleeping habits.

26. _T_ You should check your motives.

27. _T_ You should check your friendships.

MULTIPLE CHOICE: Place a check in the box next to the one, best answer to the following question:

28. What was the main good result that came to the nation of Israel after God sent them into the Babylonian Captivity for their continual sin? (1 point)

    ❏ They had the opportunity of copying and distributing the Ten Commandments to their children.

    ❏ They were able to bring out of Babylon wealth they used to rebuild the temple.

    ☑ As a nation, they never slid back into idolatry.

    ❏ As a nation, they developed a new form of writing they used in writing some of the Old Testament.

SHORT ANSWER: Answer the following questions.

29. Name three areas of your life where you believe you could become more focused. (6 points; 2 points each)

    a.

    b.   *Answer will vary.*

    c.

115

30. Explain what personal changes you could make in each area you mentioned above to help you stay focused. (6 points; 2 points each)

    a.

    b.   *Answer will vary.*

    c.

ESSAY: Answer the following question using complete sentences.

31. How might you apply the seven steps to success from the text to your own personal life? Include in your answer each of the seven steps and one application to your life for each of the steps. (14 points; 2 points each)

    Life applications will vary but the seven steps should be included which are:

    1. *Make wise decisions*
       - *Learn from others' decisions*
       - *Get input from mature adults you trust*
       - *Take time to think about your decisions*
       - *Pray for wisdom*
    2. *Stay mentally focused*
    3. *Gain self-control*
    4. *Develop appropriate boundaries*
    5. *Set realistic goals*
    6. *Become a lifelong learner*
    7. *Stay motivated*

Total Health •• **Chapter 8 • Quiz A**

Unit 3: Social Health

Sections 8.1-8.2

25 Points

Name:_____

Date: _____

Score: _____

MATCHING: (9 points; 1 point each) For each numbered item, place the letter of the correct answer in the space provided at the left of each item. Each answer can be used only once.

1. _____ Communication
2. _____ Friendship
3. _____ Nonverbal communication
4. _____ Social health
5. _____ Substitutions
6. _____ Relationship
7. _____ Artificial relationships
8. _____ Wall (between people)
9. _____ Verbal communication

A. Your ability to get along with different kinds of people.

B. A social connection in which people willingly share common interests or activities.

C. A barrier between people that hinders their communication.

D. Sharing a message without talking such as body language or hand motions.

E. The act of expressing thoughts, feelings, information, or beliefs easily or effectively through speech, writing, or signs.

F. Sharing a message through words, talking.

G. Replacing one person or thing with another.

H. Bonding with someone or something that doesn't really exist as an actual living person in real life.

I. A tie with people by blood, marriage, work, or social role.

SHORT ANSWER: Answer the following questions.

10. What is the danger in substituting a 'thing' for a real person—maybe even a friendship? Give two examples of 'things' that can be replacements for friendships. (3 points)

11. Why is it that so many teens have difficulty finding the words to share how they really feel with others? (2 points)

12. What is one characteristic of two people being "best" or very close friends? (2 points)

13. Of all the friendships in your life, your relationship with whom has the potential of being the deepest and most fulfilling of all? (2 points)

14. What's meant by the phrase, "Most people can talk, but not everyone can genuinely communicate"? (2 points)

15. What is one of the two ways given in the text that tells how relationship conflicts can be resolved? (2 points)

16. List 3 of the 12 skills of good communication. (3 points total)

Total Health · Chapter 8 • Quiz A Key

Unit 3: Social Health   25 points

Sections 8.1-8.2

MATCHING: (9 points; 1 point each) For each numbered item, place the letter of the correct answer in the space provided at the left of each item. Each answer can be used only once.

1. _E_ Communication
2. _B_ Friendship
3. _D_ Nonverbal communication
4. _A_ Social health
5. _G_ Substitutions
6. _I_ Relationship
7. _H_ Artificial relationships
8. _C_ Wall (between people)
9. _F_ Verbal communication

A. Your ability to get along with different kinds of people.

B. A social connection in which people willingly share common interests or activities.

C. A barrier between people that hinders their communication.

D. Sharing a message without talking such as body language or hand motions.

E. The act of expressing thoughts, feelings, information, or beliefs easily or effectively through speech, writing, or signs.

F. Sharing a message through words, talking.

G. Replacing one person or thing with another.

H. Bonding with someone or something that doesn't really exist as an actual living person in real life.

I. A tie with people by blood, marriage, work, or social role.

SHORT ANSWER: Answer the following questions.

10. What is the danger in substituting a 'thing' for a real person—maybe even a friendship? Give two examples of 'things' that can be replacements for friendships. (3 points)

    This is dangerous because it can promote isolation and a lack of accountability with others. A computer program or game, a Hollywood actor or actress, a star athlete or the lives of those on a soap opera or sitcom can become artificial relationships for some teens.

11. Why is it that so many teens have difficulty finding the words to share how they really feel with others? (2 points)

    The electronic entertainment they watch all the time doesn't require them to put their own thoughts and feelings into real words.

12. What is one characteristic of two people being "best" or very close friends? (2 points)

share common interests, have fun together, encourage each other, don't try to change each other, are able to work through conflicts, someone you can love and trust, has your best interest in mind, won't criticize or reject you for who you are, be interested in your personal, spiritual growth

13. Of all the friendships in your life, your relationship with whom has the potential of being the deepest and most fulfilling of all? (2 points)

your relationship with God

14. What's meant by the phrase, "Most people can talk, but not everyone can genuinely communicate"? (2 points)

People can use words but not necessarily really hear and understand what another person is saying.

15. What is one of the two ways given in the text that tells how relationship conflicts can be resolved? (2 points)

Learn how to express your feelings truthfully and lovingly to the other person; increase your ability to understand the other person's feelings.

16. List 3 of the 12 skills of good communication. (3 points total)
   - *Realize that first impressions can be misleading.*
   - *Choose the right time and place.*
   - *Know what your true feelings are and stick to them.*
   - *Avoid yelling, screaming, and name-calling.*
   - *Be an active and sensitive listener.*
   - *Be quick to apologize.*
   - *Accept the person even if you reject the idea.*
   - *Recognize walls in yourself and others.*
   - *Use "I" statements instead of "You" statements.*
   - *Describe the present situation only. Avoid statements that use the words "never" or "always".*
   - *Accept the fact that some conflicts will take time to be resolved.*
   - *Put yourself in the other person's place.*

Total Health ·························· Chapter 8 • Quiz B

Unit 3: Social Health

Sections 8.3-8.5

30 Points

Name:_____

Date: _____

Score: _____

MATCHING: (9 points; 1 point each) For each numbered item, place the letter of the correct answer in the space provided at the left of each item. Each answer can be used only once.

1. _____ Disrespect

2. _____ Positive peer pressure

3. _____ Revenge

4. _____ Empathy

5. _____ Reputation

6. _____ Forgiveness

7. _____ Negative peer pressure

8. _____ Respect

9. _____ Infatuation

A. What people think of you.

B. Esteem, admiration, acceptance, or courtesy; not intruding upon or interfering with another person's rights.

C. Release all of your desire to punish or get even with those who have hurt or offended you.

D. Feeling strong emotional attraction to a person of the opposite sex.

E. Wanting to get even with someone.

F. When you really feel for a person who is hurt because you've experienced the same hurt.

G. Lack of courtesy, rude or insulting; sarcastic, sassy.

H. What you feel when others encourage you to do something that is harmful for you.

I. What you feel when others encourage you to do something that is good for you.

YES OR NO: (4 points total; $^1/_2$ point each) Put a Y for Yes and a N for No as to how the statements below answer the following question:

10. Is this a healthy and mature way of acting around a person of the opposite sex?

    a. _____ Showing off to them

    b. _____ Feeling insecure and embarrassed around them

    c. _____ Being oneself; feeling relaxed

    d. _____ Treating them as a Christian brother or sister

    e. _____ Putting them down; making fun of them

    f. _____ Showing them kindness and courtesy

    g. _____ Teasing them a lot

    h. _____ Not sharing their secrets

TRUE OR FALSE: (4 points total; $^1/_2$ point each) Put a T for true or an F for false in front of the following statements:

11. _____ When you allow yourself to get deeply or emotionally attached to someone of the opposite sex and you're not ready to make a commitment, it will lead to pain and heartbreak.

12. _____ The real purpose for single dating is just having fun.

13. _____ A sign of being mature is being able to say "No" without feeling guilty.

14. _____ It is a sign of immaturity to be open to adult input when you're a mature teenager.

15. _____ It's normal to feel a need for attention.

16. _____ It's normal to want others to like you if you don't feel totally loved and accepted by your own family.

17. _____ "Courting" is an old-fashioned dating concept from which we can learn very little.

18. _____ Infatuation doesn't have a dark side. It's always fun, innocent, and healthy.

MULTIPLE CHOICE:

19. Place a check in each box below that gives a good reason (from the text) as to why your peers usually aren't the best source of advice or direction for your life: (3 points; 1 point each)

❏ Because your peers are probably struggling with the same things as you are.

❏ Because your peers don't know the different members of your family.

❏ Because your peers lack personal experience and can't give practical advice.

❏ Because your peers often cannot keep secrets.

20. Place a check in the box of whatever statement(s) are good ways for developing a great reputation. (4 points total; 1 point each)

❏ Look for ways to help others.

❏ Don't practice what you preach.

❏ Be friendly to everyone.

❏ Keep your word.

❏ Share secrets.

❏ Defend your friends.

21. Place a check by *the one* definition of the meaning of true forgiveness. True forgiveness is... (2 points)

❏ Never telling anyone else who hurt you.

❏ Forgetting how the person hurt you.

❏ Releasing the person from your judgment.

❏ Avoiding the person in the future.

❏ Praying for the person who hurt you to be judged by God.

❏ Whenever it comes, simply pushing the hurt of the past out of your mind.

SHORT ANSWER: Answer the following questions.

22. How can a person avoid negative peer pressure? (2 points)

23. The Bible condemns partiality or favoritism. Read James 2:1-13 and explain how this principle can be applied to your life today. (2 points)

Total Health ···················· Chapter 8 • Quiz B Key

Unit 3: Social Health

Sections 8.3-8.5

30 points

MATCHING: (9 points; 1 point each) For each numbered item, place the letter of the correct answer in the space provided at the left of each item. Each answer can be used only once.

1. __G__ Disrespect
2. __I__ Positive peer pressure
3. __E__ Revenge
4. __F__ Empathy
5. __A__ Reputation
6. __C__ Forgiveness
7. __H__ Negative peer pressure
8. __B__ Respect
9. __D__ Infatuation

A. What people think of you.

B. Esteem, admiration, acceptance, or courtesy; not intruding upon or interfering with another person's rights.

C. Release all of your desire to punish or get even with those who have hurt or offended you.

D. Feeling strong emotional attraction to a person of the opposite sex.

E. Wanting to get even with someone.

F. When you really feel for a person who is hurt because you've experienced the same hurt.

G. Lack of courtesy, rude or insulting; sarcastic, sassy.

H. What you feel when others encourage you to do something that is harmful for you.

I. What you feel when others encourage you to do something that is good for you.

YES OR NO: (4 points total; $^1/_2$ point each) Put a Y for Yes and a N for No as to how the statements below answer the following question:

10. Is this a healthy and mature way of acting around a person of the opposite sex?

    a. __N__ Showing off to them

    b. __N__ Feeling insecure and embarrassed around them

    c. __Y__ Being oneself; feeling relaxed

    d. __Y__ Treating them as a Christian brother or sister

    e. __N__ Putting them down; making fun of them

    f. __Y__ Showing them kindness and courtesy

    g. __N__ Teasing them a lot

    h. __Y__ Not sharing their secrets

TRUE OR FALSE: (4 points total; $^1/_2$ point each) Put a T for true or an F for false in front of the following statements:

11. __T__ When you allow yourself to get deeply or emotionally attached to someone of the opposite sex and you're not ready to make a commitment, it will lead to pain and heartbreak.

12. __F__ The real purpose for single dating is just having fun.

13. __T__ A sign of being mature is being able to say "No" without feeling guilty.

14. __F__ It is a sign of immaturity to be open to adult input when you're a mature teenager.

15. __T__ It's normal to feel a need for attention.

16. __T__ It's normal to want others to like you if you don't feel totally loved and accepted by your own family.

17. __F__ "Courting" is an old-fashioned dating concept from which we can learn very little.

18. __F__ Infatuation doesn't have a dark side. It's always fun, innocent, and healthy.

MULTIPLE CHOICE:

19. Place a check in each box below that gives a good reason (from the text) as to why your peers usually aren't the best source of advice or direction for your life: (3 points; 1 point each)

    ☑ Because your peers are probably struggling with the same things as you are.

    ❏ Because your peers don't know the different members of your family.

    ☑ Because your peers lack personal experience and can't give practical advice.

    ☑ Because your peers often cannot keep secrets.

20. Place a check in the box of whatever statement(s) are good ways for developing a great reputation. (4 points total; 1 point each)

    ☑ Look for ways to help others.

    ❏ Don't practice what you preach.

    ☑ Be friendly to everyone.

    ☑ Keep your word.

    ❏ Share secrets.

    ☑ Defend your friends.

21. Place a check by *the one* definition of the meaning of true forgiveness. True forgiveness is... (2 points)

    ❏ Never telling anyone else who hurt you.

    ❏ Forgetting how the person hurt you.

    ☑ Releasing the person from your judgment.

    ❏ Avoiding the person in the future.

    ❏ Praying for the person who hurt you to be judged by God.

    ❏ Whenever it comes, simply pushing the hurt of the past out of your mind.

SHORT ANSWER: Answer the following questions.

22. How can a person avoid negative peer pressure? (2 points)

    Develop good communication skills with your parents and mature, safe adults. When you invest in healthy friendships, you surround yourself with the positive influence of good friends. As a result, negative peer pressure won't affect you as much.

23. The Bible condemns partiality or favoritism. Read James 2:1-13 and explain how this principle can be applied to your life today. (2 points)

    When a teen shows favoritism only to those who look good, wear designer clothes, have money, are intelligent, have athletic ability or a cool car, they are showing partiality. God wants us to show unconditional respect to all people, Christian and non-Christian. God made each person in His image and for His own special purpose.

Total Health · Chapter 8 • Test

Unit 3: Social Health

100 Points

Name:_____

Date: _____

Score: _____

MATCHING: (9 points; 1 point each): For each numbered item, place the letter of the correct answer in the space provided at the left of each item. Each answer can be used only once.

1. _____ Communication
2. _____ Friendship
3. _____ Nonverbal communication
4. _____ Social health
5. _____ Substitutions
6. _____ Relationship
7. _____ Artificial relationships
8. _____ Walls (between people)
9. _____ Verbal communication

A. A social connection in which people willingly share common interests or activities.

B. Replacing one person or thing with another.

C. A barrier between people that hinders their communication.

D. Sharing a message without talking such as body language or hand motions.

E. Sharing a message through words, talking.

F. Bonding with someone or something that doesn't really exist as an actual living person in real life.

G. The act of expressing thoughts, feelings, information, or beliefs easily or effectively through speech, writing, or signs.

H. Your ability to get along with different kinds of people.

I. A tie with people by blood, marriage, work, or social role.

SHORT ANSWER: Answer the following questions.

10. What's meant by the phrase, "Most people can talk, but not everyone can genuinely communicate"? (2 points)

11. What is one main reason why so many teens have difficulty finding the words to share how they really feel with others? (2 points)

12. What is one of the two ways given in the text that tells how relationship conflicts can be resolved? (2 points)

13. What are three characteristics of two people being "best" or very close friends? (3 points)

14. Of all the friendships in your life, what relationship has the potential of being the deepest and most fulfilling of all? (2 points)

TRUE OR FALSE: (8 points; 1 point each) Put a T for true and an F for false in front of the following statements:

15. _____ "Courting" is an old-fashioned dating concept from which we can learn very little.

16. _____ The real purpose for single dating is just having fun.

17. _____ Infatuation doesn't have a dark side. It's always fun, innocent and healthy.

18. _____ A sign of being mature is being able to say "No" without feeling guilty.

19. _____ It is a sign of immaturity to be open to adult input.

20. _____ When you allow yourself to get deeply or emotionally attached to someone of the opposite sex and you're not ready to make a commitment, it will lead to pain and heartbreak.

21. _____ It's normal to feel a need for attention.

22. _____ It's normal to want others to like you if you don't feel totally loved and accepted by your own family.

SHORT ANSWER: Answer the following questions.

23. List seven of the twelve skills of good communication. (7 points; 1 point each)

24. What is the danger in substituting a 'thing' for a real person—maybe even a friendship? (2 points)

25. Give two examples of 'things' that can be replacements for friendships. (4 points; 2 points each)

26. How can a person avoid negative peer pressure? (4 points)

MATCHING (9 points; 1 point each): For each numbered item, place the letter of the correct answer in the space provided at the left of each item. Each answer can be used only once.

27. _____ Disrespect
28. _____ Positive peer pressure
29. _____ Revenge
30. _____ Empathy
31. _____ Reputation
32. _____ Forgiveness
33. _____ Negative peer pressure
34. _____ Respect
35. _____ Infatuation

A. Release all of your desire to punish or get even with those who have hurt of offended you.
B. What you feel when others encourage you to do something that is good for you.
C. Feeling strong emotional attraction to a person of the opposite sex.
D. What people think of you.
E. When you really feel for a person who is hurt because you've experienced the same hurt.
F. Esteem, admiration, acceptance, or courtesy; not intruding upon or interfering with another person's rights.
G. Wanting to get even with someone.
H. Lack of courtesy, rude or insulting; sarcastic, sassy.
I. What you feel when others encourage you to do something that is harmful for you.

SHORT ANSWER: Answer the following questions.

36. List five of the thirteen ways to show respect to others, <u>and</u> list the future benefit to you for each. (10 points; 1 point each)

Courtesy	*Benefit to You*
(1)	(1)
(2)	(2)
(3)	(3)
(4)	(4)
(5)	(5)

37. List three of the six ways to develop a great reputation.(3 points)

38. List five of the eight qualities of a good friend. (5 points)

MULTIPLE CHOICE: (3 points)

39. Place a check in the box for the reasons below that best state why your peers usually aren't the best source of advice or direction for your life:
    - ❑ Because your peers are probably struggling with the same things as you are.
    - ❑ Because your peers don't know the different members of your family.
    - ❑ Because your peers lack personal experience and can't give practical advice.
    - ❑ Because your peers often cannot keep secrets.

ESSAY: Answer the following question(s) using complete sentences.

40. The Bible condemns partiality or favoritism. Read James 2:1-13 and explain how this principle can be applied to your life today. Include in your answer: (15 points; 5 points each)
    - what favoritism is:
    - ways teens show favoritism:
    - how God wants us to treat others:
    - how favoritism makes others feel (those who are less favored):
    - what a person could do to change their habit of showing favoritism:

41. Read Proverbs 11:13. (10 points)

    Do you find yourself or one of your peers, talking behind someone's back or speaking negatively about others? If you do, you or he/she may develop the reputation of being a gossip. Write a paragraph explaining the following points: (5 points each)

    • Why don't those who gossip have many friends?

    • What can a person do to help themselves overcome the temptation to gossip?

Total Health ·· Chapter 8 • Test Key

Unit 3: Social Health

100 points

MATCHING: (9 points; 1 point each): For each numbered item, place the letter of the correct answer in the space provided at the left of each item. Each answer can be used only once.

1. _G_ Communication
2. _A_ Friendship
3. _D_ Nonverbal communication
4. _H_ Social health
5. _B_ Substitutions
6. _I_ Relationship
7. _F_ Artificial relationships
8. _C_ Walls (between people)
9. _E_ Verbal communication

A. A social connection in which people willingly share common interests or activities.

B. Replacing one person or thing with another.

C. A barrier between people that hinders their communication.

D. Sharing a message without talking such as body language or hand motions.

E. Sharing a message through words, talking.

F. Bonding with someone or something that doesn't really exist as an actual living person in real life.

G. The act of expressing thoughts, feelings, information, or beliefs easily or effectively through speech, writing, or signs.

H. Your ability to get along with different kinds of people.

I. A tie with people by blood, marriage, work, or social role.

SHORT ANSWER: Answer the following questions.

10. What's meant by the phrase, "Most people can talk, but not everyone can genuinely communicate"? (2 points)

    People can use words but not necessarily really hear and understand what another person is saying.

11. What is one main reason why so many teens have difficulty finding the words to share how they really feel with others? (2 points)

    The electronic entertainment they watch all the time doesn't require them to put their own thoughts and feelings into real words.

12. What is one of the two ways given in the text that tells how relationship conflicts can be resolved? (2 points)

    Learn how to express your feelings truthfully and lovingly to the other person; increase your ability to understand the other person's feelings

13. What are three characteristics of two people being "best" or very close friends? (3 points)

    a. *share common interests*
    b. *have fun together*
    c. *encourage each other*
    d. *don't try to change each other*
    e. *are able to work through conflicts*
    f. *someone you can love and trust*
    g. *has your best interest in mind*
    h. *won't criticize or reject you for who you are*
    i. *be interested in your personal, spiritual growth*

135

14. Of all the friendships in your life, what relationship has the potential of being the deepest and most fulfilling of all? (2 points)

Your relationship with God.

TRUE OR FALSE: (8 points; 1 point each) Put a T for true and an F for false in front of the following statements:

15. _F_ "Courting" is an old-fashioned dating concept from which we can learn very little.

16. _F_ The real purpose for single dating is just having fun.

17. _F_ Infatuation doesn't have a dark side. It's always fun, innocent and healthy.

18. _T_ A sign of being mature is being able to say "No" without feeling guilty.

19. _F_ It is a sign of immaturity to be open to adult input.

20. _T_ When you allow yourself to get deeply or emotionally attached to someone of the opposite sex and you're not ready to make a commitment, it will lead to pain and heartbreak.

21. _T_ It's normal to feel a need for attention.

22. _T_ It's normal to want others to like you if you don't feel totally loved and accepted by your own family.

SHORT ANSWER: Answer the following questions.

23. List seven of the twelve skills of good communication. (7 points; 1 point each)
    a. *Realize that first impressions can be misleading.*
    b. *Choose the right time and place.*
    c. *Know what your true feelings are and stick to them.*
    d. *Avoid yelling, screaming, and name-calling.*
    e. *Be an active and sensitive listener.*
    f. *Be quick to apologize.*
    g. *Accept the person even if you reject the idea.*
    h. *Recognize walls in yourself and others.*
    i. *Use "I" statements instead of "You" statements.*
    j. *Describe the present situation only. Avoid statements that use the words "never" or "always".*
    k. *Accept the fact that some conflicts will take time to be resolved.*
    l. *Put yourself in the other person's place.*

24. What is the danger in substituting a 'thing' for a real person—maybe even a friendship? (2 points)

This is dangerous because it can promote isolation and a lack of accountability with others.

25. Give two examples of 'things' that can be replacements for friendships. (4 points; 2 points each)

A computer program or game, a Hollywood actor or actress, a star athlete or the lives of those on a soap opera or sitcom can become artificial relationships for some teens.

26. How can a person avoid negative peer pressure? (4 points)

Develop good communication skills with your parents and mature, safe adults. When you invest in healthy friendships, you surround yourself with the positive influence of good friends. As a result, negative peer pressure won't affect you as much.

MATCHING (9 points; 1 point each): For each numbered item, place the letter of the correct answer in the space provided at the left of each item. Each answer can be used only once.

27. _H_ Disrespect
28. _B_ Positive peer pressure
29. _G_ Revenge
30. _E_ Empathy
31. _D_ Reputation
32. _A_ Forgiveness
33. _I_ Negative peer pressure
34. _F_ Respect
35. _C_ Infatuation

A. Release all of your desire to punish or get even with those who have hurt of offended you.
B. What you feel when others encourage you to do something that is good for you.
C. Feeling strong emotional attraction to a person of the opposite sex.
D. What people think of you.
E. When you really feel for a person who is hurt because you've experienced the same hurt.
F. Esteem, admiration, acceptance, or courtesy; not intruding upon or interfering with another person's rights.
G. Wanting to get even with someone.
H. Lack of courtesy, rude or insulting; sarcastic, sassy.
I. What you feel when others encourage you to do something that is harmful for you.

SHORT ANSWER: Answer the following questions.

36. List five of the thirteen ways to show respect to others, <u>and</u> list the future benefit to you for each. (10 points; 1 point each)

Courtesy	*Benefit to You*
a. Holding the door for others	Politeness shows selflessness, girls like it
b. Not cutting in front of others	Putting others first will help others trust, respect you
c. Saying "Please" and "Thank you"	Others will enjoy being around you
d. Pulling the chair out for others to sit	Others will appreciate the thoughtfulness
e. Standing when adults enter the room	Others will respect you more, boss will respect you for it
f. Not interrupting others when they are speaking	Gain/keep more friends
g. Being an attentive listener	Establishes more trust, rapport with others
h. Giving firm handshakes	Makes better first impression
i. Sharing your umbrella	Shows others your thoughtfulness
j. Writing thank-you notes	Others will appreciate your thoughtfulness
k. Taking dishes to the sink	Helpfulness and volunteering when not asked shows thoughtfulness
l. Using breath mints etc.	Everyone will appreciate this
m. Keeping nails, hands clean	Others will appreciate your cleanliness

137

37. List three of the six ways to develop a great reputation.(3 points)

    a. look for ways to help   *d. keep your word*

    b. defend your friends   *e. don't gossip*

    c. be friendly to everyone   *f. love God sincerely*

38. List five of the eight qualities of a good friend. (5 points)

    a. shares the same belief in God as you

    b. encourages you to do things that are the best for you

    c. offers to pray with you about your areas of struggle

    d. encourages you to talk to your parents or other trusted adults when you're having problems

    e. shows loyalty to you by standing by you when life gets rough

    f. keeps his/her promises

    g. tells the truth

    h. sticks up for you in front of others when others try to put you down

MULTIPLE CHOICE: (3 points)

39. Place a check in the box for the reasons below that best state why your peers usually aren't the best source of advice or direction for your life:

    ☑ Because your peers are probably struggling with the same things as you are.

    ❏ Because your peers don't know the different members of your family.

    ☑ Because your peers lack personal experience and can't give practical advice.

    ☑ Because your peers often cannot keep secrets.

ESSAY: Answer the following question(s) using complete sentences.

40. The Bible condemns partiality or favoritism. Read James 2:1-13 and explain how this principle can be applied to your life today. Include in your answer: (15 points; 5 points each)

    • what favoritism is:

    • ways teens show favoritism:

    • how God wants us to treat others:

    • how favoritism makes others feel (those who are less favored):

    • what a person could do to change their habit of showing favoritism:

    Giving more attention some rather than treating all men/women equally. When a teen shows favoritism to only those who look good, wear designer clothes, have money, are intelligent, have athletic ability or have a cool car, they are showing partiality. This makes others feel less valued and contributes to their low self-esteem. God wants us to show unconditional respect to all people, Christian and non-Christian. God made each person in His image and for His own special purpose. If you had a habit of showing favoritism you could pay more attention to the less popular, unlovely, and involve others in your life. Treat all people equally. This will help change your heart.

41. Read Proverbs 11:13. (10 points)

    Do you find yourself or one of your peers, talking behind someone's back or speaking negatively about others? If you do, you or he/she may develop the reputation of being a gossip. Write a paragraph explaining the following points: (5 points each)

    • Why don't those who gossip have many friends?

    • What can a person do to help themselves overcome the temptation to gossip?

    Gossips don't have many friends except for other gossips. They can't keep their friends for very long because they don't respect other people's private matters. Ask God to help you overcome the temptation to gossip. The next time you are around friends, practice saying something nice about a person who is not with you and see what the response is in the group. Speaking positive about others is part of becoming more like Christ.

Total Health ·················· Chapter 9 • Quiz A

Unit 3: Social Health

Sections 9.1-9.4

25 Points

Name:_____

Date: _____

Score: _____

MATCHING: (15 points total; 1 point each) For each numbered item, place the letter of the correct answer in the space provided at the left of each item. Each answer can be used only once.

1. _____ Dandruff
2. _____ Acne
3. _____ Epidermis
4. _____ Keratin
5. _____ Sebum
6. _____ Subcutaneous layer
7. _____ Whitehead
8. _____ Dermatologist
9. _____ Head lice
10. _____ Follicle
11. _____ Dermis
12. _____ Blackhead
13. _____ Cuticle
14. _____ Ingrown toenail
15. _____ Pimple

A. A hard substance that gives nails their strength.

B. Occurs when the pores of your skin become clogged with oil.

C. The outer layer of skin.

D. The roots of your hair are secured in these small pockets.

E. A clogged pour that has become infected and filled with pus; the most serious type of acne.

F. The middle layer of skin.

G. A nail that pushes into the skin on the side of your toe.

H. Surrounds the nail and is made of a nonliving skin; protects the base of the nail from germs and bacteria.

I. A condition in which the outer layer of skin on the scalp flakes off.

J. A doctor who treats skin disorders.

K. A type of acne that is created when oil becomes trapped inside a pore.

L. An oily substance that eventually clogs the pores of your skin.

M. A pore that's plugged with oil but is exposed to the air.

N. The deepest layer of skin.

O. Insects that live in the hair and look very similar to dandruff.

SHORT ANSWER: Answer the following questions.

16. What is one reason as to why you should take the time to develop good habits of personal hygiene? (1 point)

17. If you get acne, what is one "don't" of caring for your skin? (1 point)

18. Since the rays of the sun have more of a powerful effect on us than they used to, what are two recommendations to protect yourself from over-exposure? (2 points)

MULTIPLE CHOICE: Place a check in the box below which is the correct answer to the question.

19. What is the largest organ of your body? (1 point)
    - ❑ Your brain
    - ❑ Your heart
    - ❑ Your skin
    - ❑ Your bones

TRUE OR FALSE: Place a T for true or a F for false in front of each statement below about your skin: (3 points; ¹/₂ point each)

20. _____ Your skin shields your body against outside germs.

21. _____ Your skin is too thin to guard your internal organs from heat or cold.

22. _____ Your skin's nerve endings help to protect you from danger.

23. _____ Your skin's nerve endings help you to enjoy food and touch.

24. _____ Your skin will respond well to any soap with which you wash it.

25. _____ Your skin is self-cleaning, so it doesn't require regular bathing.

TRUE OR FALSE: Place a T for true or a F for false in front of each statement below about your hair. (2 points; ¹/₂ point each)

26. _____ Good advice for a bad haircut is, "It'll always grow back."

27. _____ The best hairstyle for you might be different for someone else because of the difference in your hair type as well as the shape of your head and face.

28. _____ A teen should always choose a hairstyle that's "in" so that he/she can better witness for Christ.

29. _____ Your hair is strong enough to lift a car weighing one ton.

Total Health · Chapter 9 • Quiz A Key

Unit 3: Social Health   25 points

Sections 9.1-9.4

MATCHING: (15 points total; 1 point each) For each numbered item, place the letter of the correct answer in the space provided at the left of each item. Each answer can be used only once.

1. __I__ Dandruff
2. __B__ Acne
3. __C__ Epidermis
4. __A__ Keratin
5. __L__ Sebum
6. __N__ Subcutaneous layer
7. __K__ Whitehead
8. __J__ Dermatologist
9. __O__ Head lice
10. __D__ Follicle
11. __F__ Dermis
12. __M__ Blackhead
13. __H__ Cuticle
14. __G__ Ingrown toenail
15. __E__ Pimple

A. A hard substance that gives nails their strength.
B. Occurs when the pores of your skin become clogged with oil.
C. The outer layer of skin.
D. The roots of your hair are secured in these small pockets.
E. A clogged pour that has become infected and filled with pus; the most serious type of acne.
F. The middle layer of skin.
G. A nail that pushes into the skin on the side of your toe.
H. Surrounds the nail and is made of a nonliving skin; protects the base of the nail from germs and bacteria.
I. A condition in which the outer layer of skin on the scalp flakes off.
J. A doctor who treats skin disorders.
K. A type of acne that is created when oil becomes trapped inside a pore.
L. An oily substance that eventually clogs the pores of your skin.
M. A pore that's plugged with oil but is exposed to the air.
N. The deepest layer of skin.
O. Insects that live in the hair and look very similar to dandruff.

SHORT ANSWER: Answer the following questions.

16. What is one reason as to why you should take the time to develop good habits of personal hygiene? (1 point)

    Being clean and attractive will definitely enhance your looks, but try not to fall into the trap of always wanting to look good for other people.

    Taking care of yourself makes you feel good about yourself.

    Using good personal hygiene shows respect, not only to others, but also to yourself. Practicing good hygiene daily will boost your confidence in social situations and positively affect your relationships with others.

17. If you get acne, what is one "don't" of caring for your skin? (1 point)

    Don't squeeze or pick at your acne. This can cause infection and scarring.

    Don't use heavy creams or moisturizers on the affected areas.

    Don't touch your face with your hands or fingers. This can place more oil and dirt on your face.

    Don't let acne get you depressed or prevent you from having fun.

18. Since the rays of the sun have more of a powerful effect on us than they used to, what are two recommendations to protect yourself from over-exposure? (2 points)

    Use a sunscreen at all times.

    Cover up your exposed skin areas.

    Avoid the intense sun time, i.e., between 10:00AM – 3:00PM.

    Avoid using tanning beds.

MULTIPLE CHOICE: Place a check in the box below which is the correct answer to the question.

19. What is the largest organ of your body? (1 point)
    - ❏ Your brain
    - ❏ Your heart
    - ☑ Your skin
    - ❏ Your bones

TRUE OR FALSE: Place a T for true or a F for false in front of each statement below about your skin: (3 points; ¹/₂ point each)

20. _T_ Your skin shields your body against outside germs.

21. _F_ Your skin is too thin to guard your internal organs from heat or cold.

22. _T_ Your skin's nerve endings help to protect you from danger.

23. _T_ Your skin's nerve endings help you to enjoy food and touch.

24. _F_ Your skin will respond well to any soap with which you wash it.

25. _F_ Your skin is self-cleaning, so it doesn't require regular bathing.

TRUE OR FALSE: Place a T for true or a F for false in front of each statement below about your hair. (2 points; ¹/₂ point each)

26. _T_ Good advice for a bad haircut is, "It'll always grow back."

27. _T_ The best hairstyle for you might be different for someone else because of the difference in your hair type as well as the shape of your head and face.

28. _F_ A teen should always choose a hairstyle that's "in" so that he/she can better witness for Christ.

29. _T_ Your hair is strong enough to lift a car weighing one ton.

Total Health ···················· Chapter 9 • Quiz B

Unit 3: Social Health

Sections 9.5-9.7

25 Points

Name:_____

Date: _____

Score: _____

MATCHING: (15 points total; 1 point each) For each numbered item, place the letter of the correct answer in the space provided at the left of each item. Each answer can be used only once.

1. _____ Sty
2. _____ Masticate
3. _____ Pink eye
4. _____ Periodontium
5. _____ Astigmatism
6. _____ Cavity
7. _____ Nearsightedness
8. _____ Plaque
9. _____ Farsightedness
10. _____ Tartar
11. _____ Halitosis
12. _____ Gingivitis
13. _____ Periodontal disease
14. _____ Malocclusion
15. _____ Orthodontics

A. When your upper and lower teeth don't line up very well.

B. A substance that hardens on your teeth.

C. The name of the bone, tissue, and gum that support your teeth.

D. A condition where a person has difficulty seeing things that are close.

E. Bad breath.

F. When bacteria combine with sugary foods and form an acid.

G. A grainy, sticky coating that is constantly forming on your teeth.

H. Chew thoroughly.

I. A gum disease caused by a build-up of plaque and tartar on your teeth.

J. When one of the small glands in your eyelid gets infected and swollen. It may look like a pimple.

K. A very contagious condition caused by a bacterial infection.

L. More advanced gum disease.

M. Braces can treat severe irregularities.

N. A condition in which a person's vision is distorted due to the irregular shape of the cornea or lens.

O. A condition where a person has difficulty seeing things that are far away.

SHORT ANSWER: Answer the following questions.

16. List three ways to take good care of your teeth. (3 points)

17. What is the most common form of ear trouble? ($1/2$ point)

145

18. How might a person do a "posture check" on him/herself? ($^{1}/_{2}$ point)

FILL IN THE BLANK: (1 point)

19. Especially for teens, "listening to _____ can cause damage to the eardrum and result in a loss of hearing."

TRUE OR FALSE: (4 points; 1 point each) Place a T for true or a F for false in front of the following statements about good posture.

20. _____ Good posture makes you look more attractive.

21. _____ Good posture does not reflect a more positive self-image to others.

22. _____ Good posture helps you to be more alert in class.

23. _____ Good posture does not strengthen your bones or your muscles.

MULTIPLE CHOICE: (1 point)

24. Place a check in the box for the safest and most healthy way to carry your backpack full of school books.

❑ Carry the backpack over the same shoulder as you are either "right-handed" or "left-handed".

❑ Carry the backpack over the same shoulder all the time so that your body can adjust to it better.

❑ Carry the backpack evenly over both shoulders—not just slung over one of them.

Total Health · Chapter 9 • Quiz B Key

Unit 3: Social Health

25 points

Sections 9.5-9.7

MATCHING: (15 points total; 1 point each) For each numbered item, place the letter of the correct answer in the space provided at the left of each item. Each answer can be used only once.

1. _J_ Sty
2. _H_ Masticate
3. _K_ Pink eye
4. _C_ Periodontium
5. _N_ Astigmatism
6. _F_ Cavity
7. _O_ Nearsightedness
8. _G_ Plaque
9. _D_ Farsightedness
10. _B_ Tartar
11. _E_ Halitosis
12. _I_ Gingivitis
13. _L_ Periodontal disease
14. _A_ Malocclusion
15. _M_ Orthodontics

A. When your upper and lower teeth don't line up very well.
B. A substance that hardens on your teeth.
C. The name of the bone, tissue, and gum that support your teeth.
D. A condition where a person has difficulty seeing things that are close.
E. Bad breath.
F. When bacteria combine with sugary foods and form an acid.
G. A grainy, sticky coating that is constantly forming on your teeth.
H. Chew thoroughly.
I. A gum disease caused by a build-up of plaque and tartar on your teeth.
J. When one of the small glands in your eyelid gets infected and swollen. It may look like a pimple.
K. A very contagious condition caused by a bacterial infection.
L. More advanced gum disease.
M. Braces can treat severe irregularities.
N. A condition in which a person's vision is distorted due to the irregular shape of the cornea or lens.
O. A condition where a person has difficulty seeing things that are far away.

SHORT ANSWER: Answer the following questions.

16. List three ways to take good care of your teeth. (3 points)
    a. Brush your teeth after each meal.   *b. Brush your tongue.*
    c. Change your toothbrush.   *d. Floss at least once a day.*
    e. Use fluoride.   *f. Eat healthfully.*
    g. Visit your dentist twice a year.

17. What is the most common form of ear trouble? ($^1/_2$ point)
    An ear infection. A viral or bacterial infection of the nose, throat, or Eustachian tubes can cause intense ear pain. Unlike a middle ear infection, swimmer's ear occurs in the outer ear.

147

18. How might a person do a "posture check" on him/herself? ($^{1}/_{2}$ point)

When sitting down, try always to have your seat and lower back pushed back up against the back of the chair. This will help to prevent undue stress on your lower back muscles and help to prevent lower back pain. Imagine a string with a helium balloon connected to the crown (the very highest part) of your head. Pretend the balloon is pulling straight upward. Your chin should go down and your neck come back into proper alignment with your shoulders. If you still have posture problems, imagine that same string and balloon on the front of your chest pulling your chest up and out.

FILL IN THE BLANK: (1 point)

19. Especially for teens, "listening to ___*loud music*___ can cause damage to the eardrum and result in a loss of hearing."

TRUE OR FALSE: (4 points; 1 point each) Place a T for true or a F for false in front of the following statements about good posture.

20. _*T*_ Good posture makes you look more attractive.

21. _*F*_ Good posture does not reflect a more positive self-image to others.

22. _*T*_ Good posture helps you to be more alert in class.

23. _*F*_ Good posture does not strengthen your bones or your muscles.

MULTIPLE CHOICE: (1 point)

24. Place a check in the box for the safest and most healthy way to carry your backpack full of school books.

❏ Carry the backpack over the same shoulder as you are either "right-handed" or "left-handed".

❏ Carry the backpack over the same shoulder all the time so that your body can adjust to it better.

☑ Carry the backpack evenly over both shoulders—not just slung over one of them.

Total Health ························· Chapter 9 • Test

Unit 3: Social Health

100 Points

Name:_____

Date: _____

Score: _____

MATCHING (15 points total; 1 point each): For each numbered item, place the letter of the correct answer in the space provided at the left of each item. Each answer can be used only once.

1. _____ Dandruff

2. _____ Acne

3. _____ Epidermis

4. _____ Keratin

5. _____ Sebum

6. _____ Subcutaneous layer

7. _____ Whitehead

8. _____ Dermatologist

9. _____ Head lice

10. _____ Follicle

11. _____ Dermis

12. _____ Blackhead

13. _____ Cuticle

14. _____ Ingrown toenail

15. _____ Pimple

A. The roots of your hair are secured in these small pockets.

B. A type of acne that is created when oil becomes trapped inside a pore.

C. The outer layer of skin.

D. The middle layer of skin.

E. A condition in which the outer layer of skin on the scalp flakes off.

F. A clogged pour that has become infected and filled with pus; the most serious type of acne.

G. A nail that pushes into the skin on the side of your toe.

H. A doctor who treats skin disorders.

I. Surrounds the nail and is made of a nonliving skin; protects the base of the nail from germs and bacteria.

J. Occurs when the pores of your skin become clogged with oil.

K. An oily substance that eventually clogs the pores of your skin.

L. A pore that's plugged with oil but is exposed to the air.

M. A hard substance that gives nails their strength.

N. The deepest layer of skin.

O. Insects that live in the hair and look very similar to dandruff.

TRUE OR FALSE: Place a T for true or a F for false in front of each statement below about your skin: (6 points; 1 point each)

16. _____ Your skin is self-cleaning, so it doesn't require regular bathing.

17. _____ Your skin shields your body against outside germs.

18. _____ Your skin's nerve endings help you to enjoy food and touch.

19. _____ Your skin is too thin to guard your internal organs from heat or cold.

20. _____ Your skin's nerve endings help to protect you from danger.

21. _____ Your skin will respond well to any soap with which you wash it.

SHORT ANSWER: Answer the following questions.

22. Since the rays of the sun have more of a powerful effect on us than they used to, what are two recommendations to protect yourself from over-exposure? (4 points; 2 points each)

23. What are two reasons as to why you should take the time to develop good habits of personal hygiene? (2 points)

24. If you get acne, what is one "don't" of caring for your skin? (1 point)

TRUE OR FALSE: Place a T for true or a F for false in front of each statement below about your hair: (4 points; 1 point each)

25. _____ A teen should always choose a hairstyle that's "in" so that he/she can better witness for Christ.

26. _____ Good advice for a bad haircut is, "It'll always grow back."

27. _____ Your hair is strong enough to lift a car weighing one ton.

28. _____ The best hairstyle for you might be different than someone else because of the difference in your hair type as well as the shape of your head and face.

MATCHING (15 points total; 1 point each): For each numbered item, place the letter of the correct answer in the space provided at the left of each item. Each answer can be used only once.

29. _____ Sty

30. _____ Masticate

31. _____ Pink eye

32. _____ Periodontium

33. _____ Astigmatism

34. _____ Cavity

35. _____ Nearsightedness

36. _____ Plaque

37. _____ Farsightedness

38. _____ Tartar

39. _____ Halitosis

40. _____ Gingivitis

41. _____ Periodontal disease

42. _____ Malocclusion

43. _____ Orthodontics

A. When your upper and lower teeth don't line up very well.

B. A substance that hardens on your teeth.

C. The name of the bone, tissue, and gum that support your teeth.

D. A condition where a person has difficulty seeing things that are close.

E. Bad breath.

F. When bacteria combines with sugary foods and forms an acid.

G. A grainy, sticky coating that is constantly forming on your teeth.

H. Chew thoroughly.

I. A gum disease caused by a build-up of plaque and tartar on your teeth.

J. When one of the small glands in your eyelid gets infected and swollen. It may look like a pimple.

K. A very contagious condition caused by a bacterial infection.

L. More advanced gum disease.

M. Braces can treat severe irregularities.

N. A condition in which a person's vision is distorted due to the irregular shape of the cornea or lens.

O. A condition where a person has difficulty seeing things that are far away.

TRUE OR FALSE: (4 points; 1 point each) Place a T for true or a F for false in front of the following statements about good posture.

44. _____ Good posture helps you to be more alert in class.

45. _____ Good posture makes you look more attractive.

46. _____ Good posture does not reflect a more positive self-image to others.

47. _____ Good posture does not strengthen your bones or your muscles.

SHORT ANSWER: Answer the following questions.

48. How might a person do a "posture check" on him/herself? (1 point)

49. How can listening to loud music be dangerous? (1 point)

50. Place a check in the box of the one safest and most healthy way to carry your backpack full of school books. (2 points)

❏ Carry the backpack over the same shoulder as you are either "right-handed" or "left-handed".

❏ Carry the backpack over the same shoulder all the time so that your body can adjust to it better.

❏ Carry the backpack evenly over both shoulders, not just slung over one of them.

51. Label the four kinds of permanent teeth that are in your mouth and give the purpose for each kind of tooth. (8 points; $\frac{1}{2}$ point for each label, $\frac{1}{2}$ point for each purpose)

a.   *purpose:*

b.   *purpose:*

c.   *purpose:*

d.   *purpose:*

e.   *purpose:*

f.   *purpose:*

g.   *purpose:*

h.   *purpose:*

52. List three ways to take good care of your teeth. (3 points)

53. Imagine you have a friend who struggles with biting his/her nails. List three words of advice you would give to this friend to help him/her stop this habit. (3 points)

54. Label the parts of the ear. (9 points)

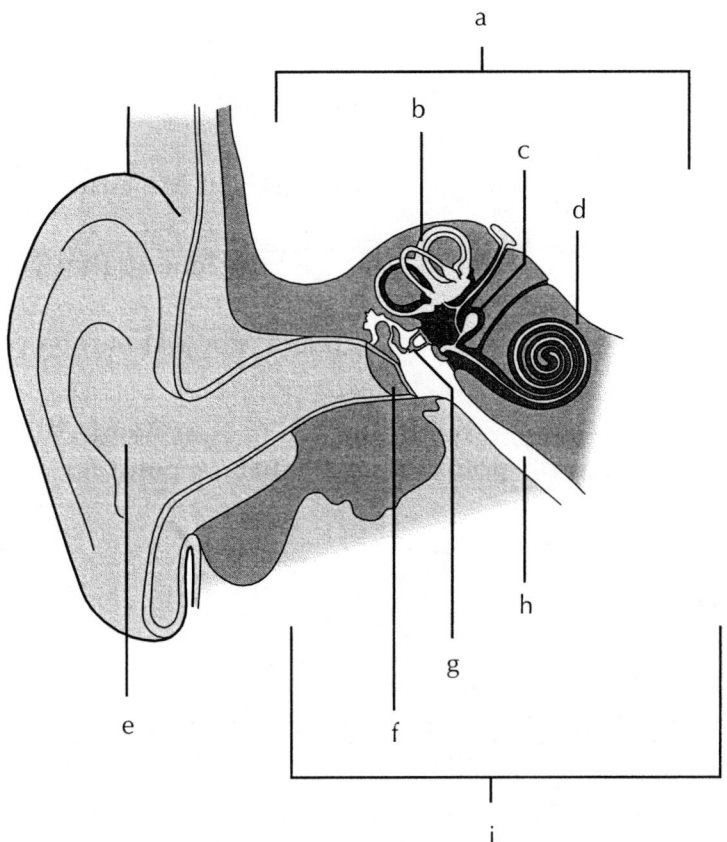

55. What is the most common form of ear trouble? (1 point)

ESSAY: Answer the following questions using complete sentences.

56. Read, "The lamp of the body is the eye. If therefore your eye is good, you whole body will be full of light." Matthew 6:22. Explain how the Bible uses this natural illustration of the eye to illustrate a spiritual truth. Include in your answer:
    - What did Jesus mean when He described your eye as the "lamp" of your body? (5 points)
    - How might this spiritual truth relate specifically to a teenager like yourself? (5 points)

57. Read Proverbs 20:12. "The hearing ear and the seeing eye; the Lord has made both of them." How might this verse apply to your responsibility to your eyes and ears? Include in your answer:
    - What examples from society do you hear and see that might negatively affect your spiritual life? (5 points)
    - How do you think that you can use your eyes and ears the most to please God? (5 points)

Total Health ···························· Chapter 9 • Test Key

Unit 3: Social Health   100 points

MATCHING (15 points total; 1 point each): For each numbered item, place the letter of the correct answer in the space provided at the left of each item. Each answer can be used only once.

1. __E__ Dandruff
2. __J__ Acne
3. __C__ Epidermis
4. __M__ Keratin
5. __K__ Sebum
6. __N__ Subcutaneous layer
7. __B__ Whitehead
8. __H__ Dermatologist
9. __O__ Head lice
10. __A__ Follicle
11. __D__ Dermis
12. __L__ Blackhead
13. __I__ Cuticle
14. __G__ Ingrown toenail
15. __F__ Pimple

A. The roots of your hair are secured in these small pockets.
B. A type of acne that is created when oil becomes trapped inside a pore.
C. The outer layer of skin.
D. The middle layer of skin.
E. A condition in which the outer layer of skin on the scalp flakes off.
F. A clogged pour that has become infected and filled with pus; the most serious type of acne.
G. A nail that pushes into the skin on the side of your toe.
H. A doctor who treats skin disorders.
I. Surrounds the nail and is made of a nonliving skin; protects the base of the nail from germs and bacteria.
J. Occurs when the pores of your skin become clogged with oil.
K. An oily substance that eventually clogs the pores of your skin.
L. A pore that's plugged with oil but is exposed to the air.
M. A hard substance that gives nails their strength.
N. The deepest layer of skin.
O. Insects that live in the hair and look very similar to dandruff.

TRUE OR FALSE: Place a T for true or a F for false in front of each statement below about your skin: (6 points; 1 point each)

16. __F__ Your skin is self-cleaning, so it doesn't require regular bathing.
17. __T__ Your skin shields your body against outside germs.
18. __T__ Your skin's nerve endings help you to enjoy food and touch.
19. __F__ Your skin is too thin to guard your internal organs from heat or cold.
20. __T__ Your skin's nerve endings help to protect you from danger.
21. __F__ Your skin will respond well to any soap with which you wash it.

SHORT ANSWER: Answer the following questions.

22. Since the rays of the sun have more of a powerful effect on us than they used to, what are two recommendations to protect yourself from over-exposure? (4 points; 2 points each)

    a. Use a sunscreen at all times.   *c. Avoid the intense sun time, between 10:00AM-3:00PM.*

    b. Cover up your exposed skin areas.   *d. Avoid using tanning beds.*

23. What are two reasons as to why you should take the time to develop good habits of personal hygiene? (2 points)

    Being clean and attractive will definitely enhance your looks, but try not to fall into the trap of always wanting to look good for other people.

    Taking care of yourself makes you feel good about yourself.

    Using good personal hygiene shows respect, not only to others, but also to yourself. Practicing good hygiene daily will boost your confidence in social situations and positively affect your relationship with others.

24. If you get acne, what is one "don't" of caring for your skin? (1 point each)

    Don't squeeze or pick at your acne. This can cause infection and scarring.

    Don't use heavy creams or moisturizers on the affected areas.

    Don't touch your face with your hands or fingers. This can place more oil and dirt on your face.

    Don't let acne get you depressed or prevent you from having fun.

TRUE OR FALSE: Place a T for true or a F for false in front of each statement below about your hair: (4 points; 1 point each)

25. _F_ A teen should always choose a hairstyle that's "in" so that he/she can better witness for Christ.

26. _T_ Good advice for a bad haircut is, "It'll always grow back."

27. _T_ Your hair is strong enough to lift a car weighing one ton.

28. _T_ The best hairstyle for you might be different than someone else because of the difference in your hair type as well as the shape of your head and face.

MATCHING (15 points total; 1 point each): For each numbered item, place the letter of the correct answer in the space provided at the left of each item. Each answer can be used only once.

29. _J_ Sty

30. _H_ Masticate

31. _K_ Pink eye

32. _C_ Periodontium

33. _N_ Astigmatism

34. _F_ Cavity

35. _O_ Nearsightedness

36. _G_ Plaque

37. _D_ Farsightedness

38. _B_ Tartar

39. _E_ Halitosis

40. _I_ Gingivitis

41. _L_ Periodontal disease

42. _A_ Malocclusion

43. _M_ Orthodontics

A. When your upper and lower teeth don't line up very well.

B. A substance that hardens on your teeth.

C. The name of the bone, tissue, and gum that support your teeth.

D. A condition where a person has difficulty seeing things that are close.

E. Bad breath.

F. When bacteria combines with sugary foods and forms an acid.

G. A grainy, sticky coating that is constantly forming on your teeth.

H. Chew thoroughly.

I. A gum disease caused by a build-up of plaque and tartar on your teeth.

J. When one of the small glands in your eyelid gets infected and swollen. It may look like a pimple.

K. A very contagious condition caused by a bacterial infection.

L. More advanced gum disease.

M. Braces can treat severe irregularities.

N. A condition in which a person's vision is distorted due to the irregular shape of the cornea or lens.

O. A condition where a person has difficulty seeing things that are far away.

TRUE OR FALSE: (4 points; 1 point each) Place a T for true or a F for false in front of the following statements about good posture.

44. _T_ Good posture helps you to be more alert in class.

45. _T_ Good posture makes you look more attractive.

46. _F_ Good posture does not reflect a more positive self-image to others.

47. _F_ Good posture does not strengthen your bones or your muscles.

SHORT ANSWER: Answer the following questions.

48. How might a person do a "posture check" on him/herself? (1 point)

When sitting down, try always to have your seat and lower back pushed back up against the back of the chair. This will help to prevent undue stress on your lower back muscles and lower back pain. Imagine a string with a helium balloon connected to the crown (the very highest part) of your head. Pretend the balloon is pulling straight upward. Your chin should go down and your neck come back into proper alignment with your shoulders. If you still have posture problems, imagine that same string and balloon on the front of your chest pulling your chest up and out.

49. How can listening to loud music be dangerous? (1 point)

It can cause damage to the eardrum and result in a loss of hearing

50. Place a check in the box of the one safest and most healthy way to carry your backpack full of school books. (2 points)

❑ Carry the backpack over the same shoulder as you are either "right-handed" or "left-handed".

❑ Carry the backpack over the same shoulder all the time so that your body can adjust to it better.

☑ Carry the backpack evenly over both shoulders, not just slung over one of them.

51. Label the four kinds of permanent teeth that are in your mouth and give the purpose for each kind of tooth. (8 points; ¹/₂ point for each label, ¹/₂ point for each purpose)

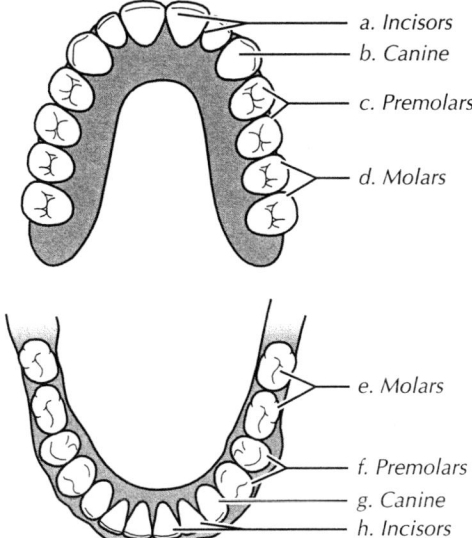

a. Incisors   *purpose: for cutting and tearing food*
b. Canine   *purpose: for tearing food*
c. Premolars   *purpose: for grinding and chewing food*
d. Molars   *purpose: for grinding and chewing food*

e. Molars   *purpose: for grinding and chewing food*

f. Premolars   *purpose: for grinding and chewing food*
g. Canine   *purpose: for tearing food*
h. Incisors   *purpose: for cutting and tearing food*

52. List three ways to take good care of your teeth. (3 points)

  a. *Brush your teeth after each meal.*   e. *Use fluoride.*

  b. *Brush your tongue.*   f. *Eat healthfully.*

  c. *Change your toothbrush.*   g. *Visit your dentist twice a year.*

  d. *Floss at least once a day.*

53. Imagine you have a friend who struggles with biting his/her nails. List three words of advice you would give to this friend to help him/her stop this habit. (3 points)

  a. *Be accountable to someone.*

  b. *Try doing something else with your hands when you feel the urge to bite your nails.*

  c. *Take note of how you feel when you want to bite your nails, then avoid that feeling or do something else when you feel that way.*

  d. *Keep your nails trimmed.*

  e. *Set goals, then treat yourself when you reach your goal of not biting your nails for a specific length of time.*

  f. *Use a bitter-tasting nail polish.*

  g. *Limit your biting to one nail.*

  h. *When you have the urge to bite your nails, talk yourself out of it.*

54. Label the parts of the ear. (9 points)

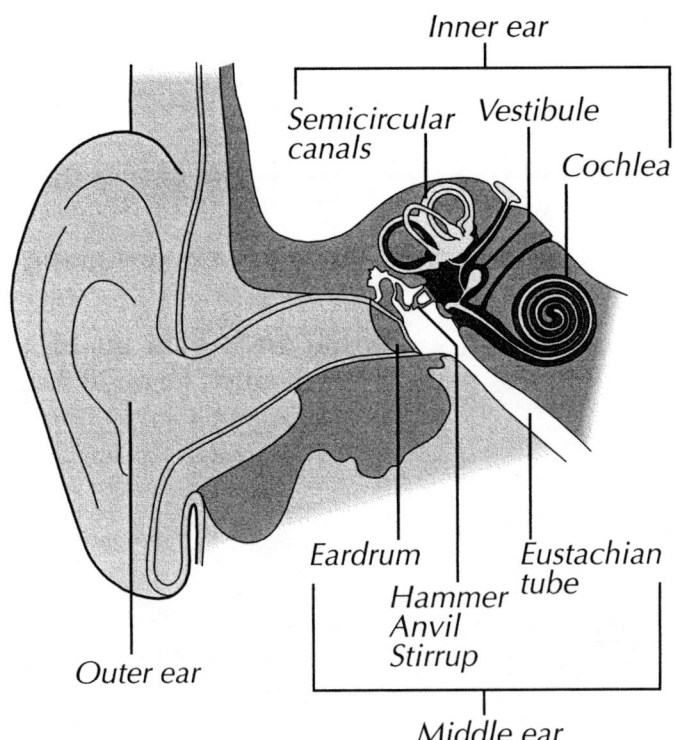

Inner ear

Semicircular canals   *Vestibule*

Cochlea

Eardrum   *Eustachian tube*

Hammer
Anvil
Stirrup

Outer ear

Middle ear

55. What is the most common form of ear trouble? (1 point)

  An ear infection. A viral or bacterial infection of the nose, throat, or Eustachian tubes can cause intense ear pain. Unlike a middle ear infection, swimmer's ear occurs in the outer ear.

ESSAY: Answer the following questions using complete sentences.

56. Read, "The lamp of the body is the eye. If therefore your eye is good, you whole body will be full of light." Matthew 6:22. Explain how the Bible uses this natural illustration of the eye to illustrate a spiritual truth. Include in your answer:

- What did Jesus mean when He described your eye as the "lamp" of your body? (5 points)
- How might this spiritual truth relate specifically to a teenager like yourself? (5 points)

  Answers may vary. The main point is that one's true inner, spiritual focus will guide one's life. E.g., my focus/goal should be more on becoming like Jesus than on sports, etc.

57. Read Proverbs 20:12. "The hearing ear and the seeing eye; the Lord has made both of them." How might this verse apply to your responsibility to your eyes and ears? Include in your answer:

- What examples from society do you hear and see that might negatively affect your spiritual life? (5 points)

  Answers vary. E.g., TV, movies, video games, internet, gambling, pornography, fame/popularity, immorality, materialism, pride, etc.

- How do you think that you can use your eyes and ears the most to please God? (5 points)

  Answers vary. E.g., read good books, listen to Christian music.

Total Health ······························· Chapter 10 • Quiz A

Unit 3: Social Health

Sections 10.1-10.3 (through p. 251)

25 Points

Name:_____

Date: _____

Score: _____

MATCHING: (20 points total; 1 point each) For each numbered item, place the letter of the correct answer in the space provided at the left of each item. Each answer can be used only once.

1. _____ MADD
2. _____ Drug abuse
3. _____ Side effects
4. _____ Addiction
5. _____ Cirrhosis
6. _____ Tolerance
7. _____ Alexander Fleming
8. _____ Alateen
9. _____ Drugs
10. _____ Stimulant
11. _____ Caffeine
12. _____ Inhibitory effect
13. _____ Withdrawal
14. _____ Alcoholism
15. _____ Alcoholics Anonymous (AA)
16. _____ Al-Anon
17. _____ Medicines
18. _____ FDA
19. _____ Prescription drug
20. _____ Nonprescription drug

A. A chronic disease of the liver that often results from a longstanding addiction to alcohol.

B. A result of alcohol that causes the blocking of the center of the brain that controls a person's degree of self-control and shyness.

C. An illness characterized by habitual, compulsive, long-term, and heavy drinking.

D. A resistance in the body to something.

E. The physical disturbance that results when an individual does not consume a substance he/she is addicted to.

F. Mothers Against Drunk Drivers.

G. A support group specifically designed for alcoholics.

H. A group designed to help children of alcoholic parents.

I. A group designed to help the husbands, wives, and friends of alcoholics.

J. Discovered the drug penicillin in London in 1928.

K. Substances that alter the function of one or more body organs.

L. Drugs that are meant to relieve pain, cure diseases, or prevent other illnesses.

M. A condition that occurs when a person uses an illegal drug or misuses a legal one.

N. Drugs that are sold only with a written order from a doctor.

O. "Over-the-counter" drugs that are medicines that can be sold without a doctor's written permission.

P. Federal Drug Administration tests drugs to make sure they are safe.

Q. Any reactions to a drug other than the intended effect.

R. A stimulant.

S. Drugs that speed up the body's nervous system.

T. A physical or mental need for a drug or other substance.

SHORT ANSWER: Answer the following questions.

21. What is God's "Freedom Formula"? (1 point)

22. List 2 immediate effects of alcohol on the body when a person drinks too much. (1 point; $\frac{1}{2}$ point each)

23. Explain the meaning of the phrase, "Advertisers don't care about your health, they only care about your money!" (1 point)

24. Explain how coffee, tea, and certain soda pop can be considered drugs. (1 point)

25. Before you decide to take your first drink, what are 2 crucial facts about alcohol that you should seriously consider? (1 point; $\frac{1}{2}$ point each)

Total Health • Chapter 10 • Quiz A Key

Unit 3: Social Health   25 points

Sections 10.1-10.3 (through p. 251)

MATCHING: (20 points total; 1 point each) For each numbered item, place the letter of the correct answer in the space provided at the left of each item. Each answer can be used only once.

1. _F_ MADD
2. _M_ Drug abuse
3. _Q_ Side effects
4. _T_ Addiction
5. _A_ Cirrhosis
6. _D_ Tolerance
7. _J_ Alexander Fleming
8. _H_ Alateen
9. _K_ Drugs
10. _S_ Stimulant
11. _R_ Caffeine
12. _B_ Inhibitory effect
13. _E_ Withdrawal
14. _C_ Alcoholism
15. _G_ Alcoholics Anonymous (AA)
16. _I_ Al-Anon
17. _L_ Medicines
18. _P_ FDA
19. _N_ Prescription drug
20. _O_ Nonprescription drug

A. A chronic disease of the liver that often results from a longstanding addiction to alcohol.

B. A result of alcohol that causes the blocking of the center of the brain that controls a person's degree of self-control and shyness.

C. An illness characterized by habitual, compulsive, long-term, and heavy drinking.

D. A resistance in the body to something.

E. The physical disturbance that results when an individual does not consume a substance he/she is addicted to.

F. Mothers Against Drunk Drivers.

G. A support group specifically designed for alcoholics.

H. A group designed to help children of alcoholic parents.

I. A group designed to help the husbands, wives, and friends of alcoholics.

J. Discovered the drug penicillin in London in 1928.

K. Substances that alter the function of one or more body organs.

L. Drugs that are meant to relieve pain, cure diseases, or prevent other illnesses.

M. A condition that occurs when a person uses an illegal drug or misuses a legal one.

N. Drugs that are sold only with a written order from a doctor.

O. "Over-the-counter" drugs that are medicines that can be sold without a doctor's written permission.

P. Federal Drug Administration tests drugs to make sure they are safe.

Q. Any reactions to a drug other than the intended effect.

R. A stimulant.

S. Drugs that speed up the body's nervous system.

T. A physical or mental need for a drug or other substance.

163

SHORT ANSWER: Answer the following questions.

21. What is God's "Freedom Formula"? (1 point)

    Show responsibility, gain more freedom; show more responsibility, gain more freedom. Freedom is earned not demanded.

22. List 2 immediate effects of alcohol on the body when a person drinks too much. (1 point; ½ point each)

    a. *Slurred speech.*

    b. *Inability to walk straight.*

    c. *Forgetfulness.*

    d. *Acting obnoxiously.*

    e. *Endangering themselves or others.*

    f. *Assaulting someone.*

    g. *Embarrassing themselves.*

23. Explain the meaning of the phrase, "Advertisers don't care about your health, they only care about your money!" (1 point)

    Advertisers promote the pleasures and 'cool' image associated with the use of tobacco, alcohol, and other products that are dangerous to your health. You don't see a commercial of a person experiencing a hangover from drinking too much.

24. Explain how coffee, tea, and certain soda pop can be considered drugs. (1 point)

    Because they are high in caffeine which is a stimulant.

25. Before you decide to take your first drink, what are 2 crucial facts about alcohol that you should seriously consider? (1 point; ½ point each)

    a. *Alcohol claims the most lives in the 15-24 year age group: 22,000 deaths per year.*

    b. *The average beginning age for alcohol consumption is 12-12.5 years old.*

    c. *The decision to drink alcohol is made two years prior to the first drink.*

    d. *Five out of seven who try alcohol will abuse it.*

    e. *One out of seven who try alcohol will become dependent, 14-17%.*

    f. *One reason alcohol abuse is such a problem is because alcohol isn't viewed as a drug, which it is. In reality, when people get drunk, they've had a drug overdose. When people are alcoholics, they have a drug addiction.*

Total Health .... Chapter 10 • Quiz B

Unit 3: Social Health

Sections 10.3 (from p. 251)-10.5

25 Points

Name:_____

Date: _____

Score: _____

MATCHING: (17 points total; 1 point each) For each numbered item, place the letter of the correct answer in the space provided at the left of each item. Each answer can be used only once.

1. _____ Depressants
2. _____ Narcotics
3. _____ Morphine and codeine
4. _____ Heroin
5. _____ PCP or angel dust
6. _____ LSD
7. _____ Hallucinogen
8. _____ Inhalants
9. _____ Denial
10. _____ Nicotine
11. _____ Tar
12. _____ Carbon monoxide
13. _____ Emphysema
14. _____ Second-hand smoke (passive smoke)
15. _____ Mainstream smoke
16. _____ Sidestream smoke
17. _____ Environmental smoke

A. The smoke that stays in the air where smokers have been smoking.

B. An irreversible lung disease that is primarily caused by smoking.

C. Refusing to acknowledge the existence of a problem.

D. A form of depressant that induces sleep or decreases feeling.

E. An extremely dangerous hallucinogen; lysergic acid diethylamide.

F. A thick, dark, sticky liquid that is formed when tobacco burns.

G. A poisonous gas that is produced by car engines and burning tobacco.

H. Drugs that tend to slow down your body's nervous system.

I. An illegal drug that is a depressant and extremely dangerous.

J. Substances whose fumes are inhaled to give the user a high-like feeling and can cause permanent brain damage.

K. A colorless, oily, water-soluble, highly toxic and addictive liquid alkaloid obtained from tobacco.

L. The smoke you inhale from another person smoking.

M. Highly addictive narcotics that are prescribed as painkillers.

N. The smoke that is inhaled and then exhaled by the smoker.

O. An extremely dangerous hallucinogen (phencyclidine).

P. A group of drugs that cause the brain to form unreal images.

Q. The smoke that comes out of the end of a lit cigarette.

SHORT ANSWER: Answer the following questions.

18. List 2 of the 9 negative effects of using marijuana. (2 points)

19. Explain the importance of not trying a drug, like marijuana, not even once. (1 point)

20. List 2 reasons why young teens still smoke even though they know it's dangerous. (2 points)

21. What is meant by the phrase, "You must 'own' your own faith?" (1 point)

TRUE OR FALSE: Place a T for true or a F for false in front of the following statements. (2 points; $^1/_2$ point each)

22. _____ God has created you with an inner desire to feel and experience His supernatural love, power, and presence.

23. _____ Instead of turning to God to meet their inner spiritual and emotional desires, some teens turn to alcohol, tobacco, drugs, sex, gangs, pornography, and non-Christian music. Those who turn to such things find deep and lasting fulfillment.

24. _____ It's not okay to feel or to experience God since our faith is not to be based at all on our feelings.

25. _____ You can personally experience part of the kingdom of God right now. You don't have to wait until you go to heaven.

Total Health ···················· Chapter 10 • Quiz B Key

Unit 3: Social Health   25 points

Sections 10.3 (from p. 251)-10.5

MATCHING: (17 points total; 1 point each) For each numbered item, place the letter of the correct answer in the space provided at the left of each item. Each answer can be used only once.

1. _H_ Depressants
2. _D_ Narcotics
3. _M_ Morphine and codeine
4. _I_ Heroin
5. _O_ PCP or angel dust
6. _E_ LSD
7. _P_ Hallucinogen
8. _J_ Inhalants
9. _C_ Denial
10. _K_ Nicotine
11. _F_ Tar
12. _G_ Carbon monoxide
13. _B_ Emphysema
14. _L_ Second-hand smoke (passive smoke)
15. _N_ Mainstream smoke
16. _Q_ Sidestream smoke
17. _A_ Environmental smoke

A. The smoke that stays in the air where smokers have been smoking.
B. An irreversible lung disease that is primarily caused by smoking.
C. Refusing to acknowledge the existence of a problem.
D. A form of depressant that induces sleep or decreases feeling.
E. An extremely dangerous hallucinogen; lysergic acid diethylamide.
F. A thick, dark, sticky liquid that is formed when tobacco burns.
G. A poisonous gas that is produced by car engines and burning tobacco.
H. Drugs that tend to slow down your body's nervous system.
I. An illegal drug that is a depressant and extremely dangerous.
J. Substances whose fumes are inhaled to give the user a high-like feeling and can cause permanent brain damage.
K. A colorless, oily, water-soluble, highly toxic and addictive liquid alkaloid obtained from tobacco.
L. The smoke you inhale from another person smoking.
M. Highly addictive narcotics that are prescribed as painkillers.
N. The smoke that is inhaled and then exhaled by the smoker.
O. An extremely dangerous hallucinogen (phencyclidine).
P. A group of drugs that cause the brain to form unreal images.
Q. The smoke that comes out of the end of a lit cigarette.

SHORT ANSWER: Answer the following questions.

18. List 2 of the 9 negative effects of using marijuana. (2 points)
   a. *Causes irregular heartbeat*
   b. *Increases hunger*
   c. *Slow down the body's rate of development*
   d. *Lowers body temperature*
   e. *Impairs perception and response time*
   f. *Damages the immune system*
   g. *Hurts the reproductive system*
   h. *Injures brain cells*
   i. *Causes the user to view reality in a distorted way*

19. Explain the importance of not trying a drug, like marijuana, not even once. (1 point)
    Just one try of a drug can cause a lifetime of addiction. Drugs today are more potent and dangerous than they were years ago. Sometimes, just one try can end in death.

20. List 2 reasons why young teens still smoke even though they know it's dangerous. (2 points)
    a. *Curiosity*
    b. *Look cool*
    c. *Peer pressure*
    d. *Want to feel a "buzz"*
    e. *Want to rebel against their parent's rules*
    f. *Think they will quit when they get older*
    g. *Feel indestructible ("I'll never get cancer.")*
    h. *"Other people smoke, and they're still living."*

21. What is meant by the phrase, "You must 'own' your own faith?" (1 point)
    To be a victorious Christian in today's culture, Christians must have their own personal convictions (strong beliefs). Christian teens cannot rely only upon what their parents believe. They must have their own personal relationship with God and begin to make their own decisions about the issues that confront them.

TRUE OR FALSE: Place a T for true or a F for false in front of the following statements. (2 points; 1/2 point each)

22. _T_ God has created you with an inner desire to feel and experience His supernatural love, power, and presence.

23. _F_ Instead of turning to God to meet their inner spiritual and emotional desires, some teens turn to alcohol, tobacco, drugs, sex, gangs, pornography, and non-Christian music. Those who turn to such things find deep and lasting fulfillment.

24. _F_ It's not okay to feel or to experience God since our faith is not to be based at all on our feelings.

25. _T_ You can personally experience part of the kingdom of God right now. You don't have to wait until you go to heaven.

Total Health • Chapter 10 • Test

Unit 3: Social Health

100 Points

Name:_____

Date: _____

Score: _____

MATCHING (20 points; 1 point each): For each numbered item, place the letter of the correct answer in the space provided at the left of each item. Each answer can be used only once.

1. _____ MADD
2. _____ Drug abuse
3. _____ Side effects
4. _____ Addiction
5. _____ Cirrhosis
6. _____ Tolerance
7. _____ Alexander Fleming
8. _____ Alateen
9. _____ Drugs
10. _____ Stimulant
11. _____ Caffeine
12. _____ Inhibitory effect
13. _____ Withdrawal
14. _____ Alcoholism
15. _____ Alcoholics Anonymous (AA)
16. _____ Al-Anon
17. _____ Medicines
18. _____ FDA
19. _____ Prescription drug
20. _____ Nonprescription drug

A. Drugs that speed up the body's nervous system.

B. A result of alcohol that causes the blocking of the center of the brain that controls a person's degree of self-control and shyness.

C. An illness characterized by habitual, compulsive, long-term, and heavy drinking.

D. A group designed to help children of alcoholic parents.

E. A resistance in the body to something.

F. Discovered the drug penicillin in London in 1928.

G. The physical disturbance that results when an individual does not consume a substance he/she is addicted to.

H. Mothers Against Drunk Driving.

I. A support group specifically designed for alcoholics.

J. A stimulant.

K. Substances that alter the function of one or more body organs.

L. Drugs that are meant to relieve pain, cure diseases, or prevent other illnesses.

M. A condition that occurs when a person uses an illegal drug or misuses a legal one.

N. A chronic disease of the liver that often results from a longstanding addiction to alcohol.

O. Federal Drug Administration tests drugs to make sure they are safe.

P. A group designed to help the husbands, wives, and friends of alcoholics.

Q. Drugs that are sold only with a written order from a doctor.

R. "Over-the-counter" drugs that are medicines that can be sold without a doctor's written permission.

S. Any reactions to a drug other than the effect intended.

T. A physical or mental need for a drug or other substance.

SHORT ANSWER: Answer the following questions.

21. Explain how coffee, tea, and certain soda pop can be considered drugs. (2 points)

169

22. Before you decide to take your first drink, what are three crucial facts about alcohol that you should seriously consider? (3 points; 1 point each)

    a.

    b.

    c.

23. Explain the meaning of the phrase, "Advertisers don't care about your health, they only care about your money!" (4 points)

MATCHING (17 points; 1 point each): For each numbered item, place the letter of the correct answer in the space provided at the left of each item. Each answer can be used only once.

24. _____ Depressants

25. _____ Narcotics

26. _____ Morphine and codeine

27. _____ Heroin

28. _____ PCP or angel dust

29. _____ LSD

30. _____ Hallucinogen

31. _____ Inhalants

32. _____ Denial

33. _____ Nicotine

34. _____ Tar

35. _____ Carbon monoxide

36. _____ Emphysema

37. _____ Second-hand smoke (passive smoke)

38. _____ Mainstream smoke

39. _____ Sidestream smoke

40. _____ Environmental smoke

A. An extremely dangerous hallucinogen (phencyclidine).

B. An irreversible lung disease that is primarily caused by smoking.

C. A thick, dark, sticky liquid that is formed when tobacco burns.

D. Drugs that tend to slow down your body's nervous system.

E. Refusing to acknowledge the existence of a problem.

F. The smoke you inhale from another person smoking.

G. Highly addictive narcotics that are prescribed as pain killers.

H. An extremely dangerous hallucinogen; lysergic acid diethylamide.

I. An illegal drug that is a depressant and is extremely dangerous.

J. A poisonous gas that is produced by car engines and burning tobacco.

K. The smoke that is inhaled and then exhaled by the smoker.

L. Substances whose fumes are inhaled to give the user a high-like feeling and can cause permanent brain damage.

M. A colorless, oily, water-soluble highly toxic and addictive, liquid alkaloid obtained from tobacco.

N. The smoke that stays in the air where smoker have been smoking.

O. A group of drugs that cause the brain to form unreal images.

P. A form of depressant that induces sleep or decreases feeling.

Q. The smoke that comes out of the end of a lit cigarette.

SHORT ANSWER: Answer the following questions.

41. List four reasons why young teens still smoke—even though they know it's dangerous. (4 points)

    a.

    b.

    c.

    d.

42. Explain the importance of not trying a drug, like marijuana, not even once. (2 points)

43. List four of the nine negative effects of using marijuana. (8 points; 2 points each)

    a.

    b.

    c.

    d.

44. How can teenagers experience part of the "kingdom of heaven" right now in their own lives? (3 points)

45. List five ways that the Bible can be practical in giving advice to teens. (5 points)
    (Receive 2 extra credit points if you can name the *one* book of the Bible from which all five ways are taken.)

    a.

    b.

    c.

    d.

    e.

ESSAY: Answer the following questions using complete sentences.

46. Explain what is meant by God's "Freedom Formula". (15 points) Include in your answer:
    - What is God's "Freedom Formula"?
    - How does this "Freedom Formula" relate to your life right now?
    - How can a teen gain more freedom?

47. What is meant by the phrase, "You must 'own' your own faith?" Include in your answer how a teen learns how to "own" his/her own faith. (10 points)

48. Imagine you have a friend who has been trying to get you to try alcohol. You really want to remain his/her friend, but you are struggling with how to handle the situation because you are feeling the pressure to give in. You are worried about your friend and want to try to convince him/her that drinking is not a good choice for either of you. (7 points)

Write a detailed response (just saying "NO" is not adequate) to your friend's comment:

"Come on! A little drink won't hurt you. I got drunk last week and it was great. Plus, everyone tries drinking at least once in his life. No one will find out. Don't be so straight!"

Total Health • Chapter 10 • Test Key

Unit 3: Social Health   100 points

MATCHING (20 points; 1 point each): For each numbered item, place the letter of the correct answer in the space provided at the left of each item. Each answer can be used only once.

1. _H_ MADD
2. _M_ Drug abuse
3. _S_ Side effects
4. _T_ Addiction
5. _N_ Cirrhosis
6. _E_ Tolerance
7. _F_ Alexander Fleming
8. _D_ Alateen
9. _K_ Drugs
10. _A_ Stimulant
11. _J_ Caffeine
12. _B_ Inhibitory effect
13. _G_ Withdrawal
14. _C_ Alcoholism
15. _I_ Alcoholics Anonymous (AA)
16. _P_ Al-Anon
17. _L_ Medicines
18. _O_ FDA
19. _Q_ Prescription drug
20. _R_ Nonprescription drug

A. Drugs that speed up the body's nervous system.
B. A result of alcohol that causes the blocking of the center of the brain that controls a person's degree of self-control and shyness.
C. An illness characterized by habitual, compulsive, long-term, and heavy drinking.
D. A group designed to help children of alcoholic parents.
E. A resistance in the body to something.
F. Discovered the drug penicillin in London in 1928.
G. The physical disturbance that results when an individual does not consume a substance he/she is addicted to.
H. Mothers Against Drunk Driving.
I. A support group specifically designed for alcoholics.
J. A stimulant.
K. Substances that alter the function of one or more body organs.
L. Drugs that are meant to relieve pain, cure diseases, or prevent other illnesses.
M. A condition that occurs when a person uses an illegal drug or misuses a legal one.
N. A chronic disease of the liver that often results from a longstanding addiction to alcohol.
O. Federal Drug Administration tests drugs to make sure they are safe.
P. A group designed to help the husbands, wives, and friends of alcoholics.
Q. Drugs that are sold only with a written order from a doctor.
R. "Over-the-counter" drugs that are medicines that can be sold without a doctor's written permission.
S. Any reactions to a drug other than the effect intended.
T. A physical or mental need for a drug or other substance.

SHORT ANSWER: Answer the following questions.

21. Explain how coffee, tea, and certain soda pop, can be considered drugs. (2 points)
    Because they are high in caffeine which is a stimulant.

22. Before you decide to take your first drink, what are three crucial facts about alcohol that you should seriously consider? (3 points; 1 point each)

    Alcohol claims the most lives in the 15-24 year age group: 22,000 deaths per year.

    a. *The average beginning age for alcohol consumption is 12-12.5 years old.*

    b. *The decision to drink alcohol is made two years prior to the first drink.*

    c. *Five out of seven who try alcohol will abuse it.*

    d. *One out of seven who try alcohol will become dependent, 14-17%.*

    e. *One reason alcohol abuse is such a problem is because alcohol isn't viewed as a drug, which it is. In reality, when people get drunk, they've had a drug overdose. When people are alcoholics, they have a drug addiction.*

23. Explain the meaning of the phrase, "Advertisers don't care about your health, they only care about your money!" (4 points)

    Advertisers promote the pleasures and 'cool' image associated with the use of tobacco, alcohol, and other products that are dangerous to your health. You don't see a commercial of a person experiencing a hangover from drinking too much.

MATCHING (17 points; 1 point each): For each numbered item, place the letter of the correct answer in the space provided at the left of each item. Each answer can be used only once.

24. _D_ Depressants

25. _P_ Narcotics

26. _G_ Morphine and codeine

27. _I_ Heroin

28. _A_ PCP or angel dust

29. _H_ LSD

30. _O_ Hallucinogen

31. _L_ Inhalants

32. _E_ Denial

33. _M_ Nicotine

34. _C_ Tar

35. _J_ Carbon monoxide

36. _B_ Emphysema

37. _F_ Second-hand smoke (passive smoke)

38. _K_ Mainstream smoke

39. _Q_ Sidestream smoke

40. _N_ Environmental smoke

A. An extremely dangerous hallucinogen (phencyclidine).

B. An irreversible lung disease that is primarily caused by smoking.

C. A thick, dark, sticky liquid that is formed when tobacco burns.

D. Drugs that tend to slow down your body's nervous system.

E. Refusing to acknowledge the existence of a problem.

F. The smoke you inhale from another person smoking.

G. Highly addictive narcotics that are prescribed as pain killers.

H. An extremely dangerous hallucinogen; lysergic acid diethylamide.

I. An illegal drug that is a depressant and is extremely dangerous.

J. A poisonous gas that is produced by car engines and burning tobacco.

K. The smoke that is inhaled and then exhaled by the smoker.

L. Substances whose fumes are inhaled to give the user a high-like feeling and can cause permanent brain damage.

M. A colorless, oily, water-soluble highly toxic and addictive, liquid alkaloid obtained from tobacco.

N. The smoke that stays in the air where smoker have been smoking.

O. A group of drugs that cause the brain to form unreal images.

P. A form of depressant that induces sleep or decreases feeling.

Q. The smoke that comes out of the end of a lit cigarette.

SHORT ANSWER: Answer the following questions.

41. List four reasons why young teens still smoke—even though they know it's dangerous. (4 points)

    a. *Curiosity*

    b. *Look cool*

    c. *Peer pressure*

    d. *Want to feel a "buzz"*

    e. *Want to rebel against their parents' rules*

    f. *Think they will quit when they get older*

    g. *Feel indestructible ("I'll never get cancer.")*

    h. *"Other people smoke and they're still living."*

42. Explain the importance of not trying a drug, like marijuana, not even once. (2 points)

    Just one try of a drug can cause a lifetime of addiction. Drugs today are more potent and dangerous than they were years ago. Sometimes, just one try can end in death.

43. List four of the nine negative effects of using marijuana. (8 points; 2 points each)

    a. *Causes irregular heartbeat*

    b. *Increases hunger*

    c. *Slows down the body's rate of development*

    d. *Lowers body temperature*

    e. *Impairs perception and response time*

    f. *Damages the immune system*

    g. *Hurts the reproductive system*

    h. *Injures brain cells*

    i. *Distorts reality*

44. How can teenagers experience part of the "kingdom of heaven" right now in their own lives? (3 points)

    By personally feeling/experiencing His presence, love, joy, peace, and power;

    By being aware of their need for God.

45. List five ways that the Bible can be practical in giving advice to teens. (5 points)

    (Receive 2 extra credit points if you can name the *one* book of the Bible from which all five ways are taken.)

    The Bible gives such practical ideas as how to:

    a. *Avoid an argument with your parents (Proverbs 17:14);*

    b. *Have lots of friends (Proverbs 18:24);*

    c. *Earn money for a bike or car (Proverbs 10:4-6);*

    d. *Choose the best boyfriend (Proverbs 22:24);*

    e. *Choose the best girlfriend (Proverbs 19:14; 31:10-31).*

ESSAY: Answer the following questions using complete sentences.

46. Explain what is meant by God's "Freedom Formula". (15 points) Include in your answer:
    - What is God's "Freedom Formula"?
    - How does this "Freedom Formula" relate to your life right now?
    - How can a teen gain more freedom?
    - *Show responsibility, gain more freedom; show more responsibility, gain more freedom.*
    - *Teens want more freedom because they are going through many changes that bring them into their own independence and personal responsibilities.*
    - *Freedom is earned, not demanded.*

47. What is meant by the phrase, "You must 'own' your own faith?" Include in your answer how a teen learns how to "own" his/her own faith. (10 points)

    To be a victorious Christian in today's culture, Christians must have their own personal convictions (strong beliefs). Christian teens cannot rely only upon what their parents believe. They must have their own personal relationship with God and begin to make their own decisions about the issues that confront them.

48. Imagine you have a friend who has been trying to get you to try alcohol. You really want to remain his/her friend, but you are struggling with how to handle the situation because you are feeling the pressure to give in. You are worried about your friend and want to try to convince him/her that drinking is not a good choice for either of you. (7 points)

Write a detailed response (just saying "NO" is not adequate) to your friend's comment:

"Come on! A little drink won't hurt you. I got drunk last week and it was great. Plus, everyone tries drinking at least once in his life. No one will find out. Don't be so straight!"

Answers will vary but may include:

· *Some of the harmful effects of alcohol.*

· *The danger of addiction.*

· *Just because no one will find out does not make it right. What about what God thinks?*

· *What have my own parents taught me about drinking? Would we be disobeying?*

· *No matter what the teens feel about drinking alcohol, they are still under age and that makes drinking illegal.*

Total Health · Chapter 11 • Quiz A

Unit 4: Spiritual Health

Sections 11.1-11.2

25 Points

Name:_____

Date: _____

Score: _____

CORRECT OR INCORRECT: (2 points; 1 point each) Place a C for "correctly used" or an I for "incorrectly used" in front of the following statements as they relate to the use of the word "comprehension".

1. _____ Gary's car started to have problems due to a quick decrease in the comprehension in the engine.

2. _____ When Katy listened to the preacher on the radio, her comprehension of some of his points was not that good because he was using words that were too big for her.

MATCHING: (5 points total; 1 point each) For each numbered item, place the letter of the correct answer in the space provided at the left of each item. Each answer can be used only once.

3. _____ Martin Luther, church reformer

4. _____ John Calvin, church reformer

5. _____ John Wycliffe, church reformer, Bible translator

6. _____ Charles Finney, evangelist

7. _____ John Wesley, founder of Methodism

A. How can true revival be maintained?

B. Doesn't the Bible say that we are saved by faith and not by works?

C. What kind of method can we use to teach Christians to be holy and disciplined?

D. Why can't I translate the Bible into the language of the common man?

E. How does the biblical doctrine of God's sovereignty apply to our daily lives?

SHORT ANSWER: Answer the following question.

8. One of the foundations to all of your leadership skills is your reading and comprehension. List 3 things you can do in order to increase your reading skills. (3 points; 1 point each)

   a.

   b.

   c.

TRUE OR FALSE: (4 points; 1 point each) Place a T for true or a F for false in front of the statements below concerning the place of questions in your life.

9. _____ It's bad to ask questions because people don't like me if I do.

10. _____ It's okay to ask questions because that's the way that I develop my God-given thinking skills.

11. _____ Too many teens allow their minds to turn into non-thinking vegetables because they spend too much time in front of electronic media.

12. _____ The human mind can be used to make inventions and discoveries—both good and bad.

LEADERS OR FOLLOWERS: (6 points; 1 point each) Place L for leaders or F for followers in front of the following statements as to which they best describe.

13. _____ Use their minds to think.

14. _____ Use most of their time "vegging out" with electronic entertainment.

15. _____ Ask good questions.

16. _____ Control their TV and movie time.

17. _____ Read interesting books.

18. _____ Aren't interested in reading, thinking or writing.

TRUE OR FALSE: (5 points; 1 point each) Place a T for true or a F for false in front of the following statements as they pertain to being good ways to develop the mind that God has given to you.

19. _____ Doing your homework before you watch TV.

20. _____ Trying to reduce the amount of time you spend thinking upon what you're reading so that you can get through the book as fast as possible.

21. _____ Criticizing the TV shows and movies you watch.

22. _____ Writing in a personal diary or journal.

23. _____ Riding your bike or talking to a friend instead of playing a computer game.

Total Health ⋯⋯⋯⋯⋯⋯⋯⋯⋯⋯ Chapter 11 • Quiz A Key

Unit 4: Spiritual Health   25 points
Sections 11.1-11.2

CORRECT OR INCORRECT: (2 points; 1 point each) Place a C for "correctly used" or an I for "incorrectly used" in front of the following statements as they relate to the use of the word "comprehension".

1. _I_ Gary's car started to have problems due to a quick decrease in the comprehension in the engine.

2. _C_ When Katy listened to the preacher on the radio, her comprehension of some of his points was not that good because he was using words that were too big for her.

MATCHING: (5 points total; 1 point each) For each numbered item, place the letter of the correct answer in the space provided at the left of each item. Each answer can be used only once.

3. _B_ Martin Luther, church reformer
4. _E_ John Calvin, church reformer
5. _D_ John Wycliffe, church reformer, Bible translator
6. _A_ Charles Finney, evangelist
7. _C_ John Wesley, founder of Methodism

A. How can true revival be maintained?
B. Doesn't the Bible say that we are saved by faith and not by works?
C. What kind of method can we use to teach Christians to be holy and disciplined?
D. Why can't I translate the Bible into the language of the common man?
E. How does the biblical doctrine of God's sovereignty apply to our daily lives?

SHORT ANSWER: Answer the following question.

8. One of the foundations to all of your leadership skills is your reading and comprehension. List 3 things you can do in order to increase your reading skills. (3 points; 1 point each)

   a. *The next time you watch a movie, look at the credits and see what book the movie was taken from. Read the book upon which your favorite movie was based. Compare the book with the movie.*

   b. *Tell yourself that you're going to spend just as much time reading as you do watching TV or movies.*

   c. *Try not using any electronic entertainment for a day, a week, or more. See if you get better grades, develop more friendship, have fun learning something new, or get more good books read.*

   d. *Find a friend who likes to read the same kind of books as you do.*

   e. *Use a Bible translation that you really understand and like.*

   f. *Help to put together a home environment that is favorable to reading.*

TRUE OR FALSE: (4 points; 1 point each) Place a T for true or a F for false in front of the statements below concerning the place of questions in your life.

9. _F_ It's bad to ask questions because people don't like me if I do.

10. _T_ It's okay to ask questions because that's the way that I develop my God-given thinking skills.

11. __T__ Too many teens allow their minds to turn into non-thinking vegetables because they spend too much time in front of electronic media.

12. __T__ The human mind can be used to make inventions and discoveries—both good and bad.

LEADERS OR FOLLOWERS: (6 points; 1 point each) Place L for leaders or F for followers in front of the following statements as to which they best describe.

13. __L__ Use their minds to think.

14. __F__ Use most of their time "vegging out" with electronic entertainment.

15. __L__ Ask good questions.

16. __L__ Control their TV and movie time.

17. __L__ Read interesting books.

18. __F__ Aren't interested in reading, thinking or writing.

TRUE OR FALSE: (5 points; 1 point each) Place a T for true or a F for false in front of the following statements as they pertain to being good ways to develop the mind that God has given to you.

19. __T__ Doing your homework before you watch TV.

20. __F__ Trying to reduce the amount of time you spend thinking upon what you're reading so that you can get through the book as fast as possible.

21. __T__ Criticizing the TV shows and movies you watch.

22. __T__ Writing in a personal diary or journal.

23. __T__ Riding your bike or talking to a friend instead of playing a computer game.

Total Health ···································· Chapter 11 • Quiz B

Unit 4: Spiritual Health

Sections 11.3-11.4

25 Points

Name:_____

Date: _____

Score: _____

MATCHING: (5 points total; 1 point each) For each numbered item, place the letter of the correct answer in the space provided at the left of each item. Each answer can be used only once.

1. _____ Intellectual

2. _____ Humility

3. _____ Countenance

4. _____ Hypocrites

5. _____ Regress

A. The expression on your face.

B. Mental; having to do with your mind.

C. To go backwards.

D. "Two-faced"; giving the impression that you have certain beliefs or feelings that you really don't have.

E. Realizing your own limitations.

SHORT ANSWER: Answer the following questions.

6. List 3 ways to show respect to your parent(s)—or to anyone. (3 points)

    a.

    b.

    c.

7. If asking questions is good, when does it become wrong or bad? (1 point)

8. What does it mean to allow your parents to "save face"? (1 point)

9. Why is this a sign of respect? (1 point)

TRUE OR FALSE: (4 points; 1 point each) Place a T for true or a F for false in front of each of the following statements as they relate to the subject of questions.

10. _____ God feels insecure and threatened whenever you ask Him a question.

11. _____ There are not that many questions in the Bible.

12. _____ God rejected people in the Scriptures whenever they asked Him a question.

13. _____ Jesus used questions to cause people to think when He taught them.

Total Health •••••••••••••••••••••••••••••••••• **Chapter 11 • Quiz B Key**

Unit 4: Spiritual Health   15 points

Sections 11.3-11.4

MATCHING: (5 points total; 1 point each) For each numbered item, place the letter of the correct answer in the space provided at the left of each item. Each answer can be used only once.

1. __B__ Intellectual   A. The expression on your face.
2. __E__ Humility   B. Mental; having to do with your mind.
3. __A__ Countenance   C. To go backwards.
4. __D__ Hypocrites   D. "Two-faced"; giving the impression that you have certain
5. __C__ Regress   beliefs or feelings that you really don't have.
                            E. Realizing your own limitations.

SHORT ANSWER: Answer the following questions.

6. List 3 ways to show respect to your parent(s)—or to anyone. (3 points)

   a. *Look at them when they're talking to you.*

   b. *Acknowledge what they've said to you by repeating it back to them or saying, for example, "Yes, Mom."*

   c. *Ask them to reconsider by giving them a good reason if you are struggling with what they've just asked you to do.*

   d. *Saying "Please" more often.*

   e. *Showing a grateful spirit by saying "Thank you" more often.*

7. If asking questions is good, when does it become wrong or bad? (1 point)

   Questions are good as long as they come from a heart that is simply seeking the truth. An attitude of pride, trying to be obnoxious or trying to make someone be embarrassed or "look bad" are ways that questioning can be wrong. Check your motives and the timing of when to ask what question.

8. What does it mean to allow your parents to "save face"? (1 point)

   Not exposing their weaknesses in front of others.

187

9. Why is this a sign of respect? (1 point)

    One of the ways that you can show respect for your parents is in allowing them to "save face". As you mature, you're going to make some mistakes and so are your parents. Your parents have a lot of pressure on them to "be right" and "do right" most of the time. Because of this pressure, they usually won't appreciate it if you expose their mistakes in a direct or disrespectful way; some won't like it at all. But, as you get older, you're going to see legitimate problems in your parents. The fact is that everybody has weaknesses because we're all fallen and broken human beings.

TRUE OR FALSE: (4 points; 1 point each) Place a T for true or a F for false in front of each of the following statements as they relate to the subject of questions.

10. _F_ God feels insecure and threatened whenever you ask Him a question.

11. _F_ There are not that many questions in the Bible.

12. _F_ God rejected people in the Scriptures whenever they asked Him a question.

13. _T_ Jesus used questions to cause people to think when He taught them.

Total Health •• Chapter 11 • Test

Unit 4: Spiritual Health

100 Points

Name:_____

Date: _____

Score: _____

TRUE OR FALSE: Place a T for true or a F for false in front of the statements below concerning the place of questions in your life. (4 points; 1 points each)

1. _____ Too many teens allow their minds to turn into non-thinking vegetables because they spend too much time in front of electronic media.

2. _____ It's bad to ask questions because people don't like me if I do.

3. _____ The human mind can be used to make inventions and discoveries—both good and bad.

4. _____ It's okay to ask questions because that's the way that I develop my God-given thinking skills.

MATCHING (5 points; 1 points each): For each numbered item, place the letter of the correct answer in the space provided at the left of each item. Each answer can be used only once.

5. _____ Martin Luther, church reformer

6. _____ John Calvin, church reformer

7. _____ John Wycliffe, church reformer, Bible translator

8. _____ Charles Finney, evangelist

9. _____ John Wesley, founder of Methodism

A. What kind of method can we use to teach Christians to be holy and disciplined?

B. How can true revival be maintained?

C. Doesn't the Bible say that we are saved by faith and not by works?

D. Why can't I translate the Bible into the language of the common man?

E. How does the biblical doctrine of God's sovereignty apply to our daily lives?

LEADERS OR FOLLOWERS: Place L for leaders or F for followers in front of the following statements as to which they best describe. (12 points; 2 points each)

10. _____ Ask good questions.

11. _____ Control their TV and movie time.

12. _____ Use most of their time "vegging out" with electronic entertainment.

13. _____ Read interesting books.

14. _____ Use their minds to think.

15. _____ Aren't interested in reading, thinking or writing.

TRUE OR FALSE: (2 points; 1 point each) Place a C for "correctly used" or an I for "incorrectly used" in front of the following statements as they relate to the use of the word "comprehension".

16. _____ Gary's car started to have problems due to a quick decrease in the comprehension in the engine.

17. _____ When Katy listened to the preacher on the radio, she was not able to comprehend some of his points because he was using words that were too big for her.

TRUE OR FALSE: Place a T for true or a F for false in front of the following statements as they pertain to being good ways to develop the mind that God has given to you. (5 points; 1 point each)

18. _____ Writing in a personal diary or journal.

19. _____ Criticizing the TV shows and movies you watch.

20. _____ Trying to reduce the amount of time you spending thinking upon what you're reading so that you can get through the book as fast as possible.

21. _____ Doing your homework before you watch TV.

22. _____ Riding your bike or talking to a friend instead of playing a computer game.

MATCHING: For each numbered item, place the letter of the correct answer in the space provided at the left of each item. Each answer can be used only once. (10 points; 2 points each)

23. _____ Humility

24. _____ Hypocrites

25. _____ Countenance

26. _____ Intellectual

27. _____ Regress

A. Mental; having to do with your mind.

B. "Two-faced"; giving the impression that you have certain beliefs or feelings that you really don't have.

C. The expression on your face.

D. To go backwards.

E. Realizing your own limitations.

TRUE OR FALSE: Place a T for true or a F for false in front of each of the following statements as they relate to the subject of questions. (8 points; 2 points each)

28. _____ There are not that many questions in the Bible.

29. _____ God feels insecure and threatened whenever you ask Him a question.

30. _____ God rejected people in the Scriptures whenever they asked Him a question.

31. _____ Jesus used questions to cause people to think when He taught them.

SHORT ANSWER: Answer the following questions.

32. One of the foundations to all of your leadership skills is your reading and comprehension. List four things you can do in order to increase your reading skills. (8 points; 2 points each)

    a.

    b.

    c.

    d.

33. What does it mean to allow your parents to "save face"? Why is this a sign of respect? (5 points)

34. If asking questions is good, when does it become wrong or bad? (4 points)

35. Thinking biblically and asking intelligent questions are signs of the following three good, biblical qualities: (3 points)

    a.

    b.

    c.

36. What four books in the Bible are considered the Wisdom Books? (4 points)

    a.

    b.

    c.

    d.

37. List three ways to show respect to your parent(s)—or to anyone. (6 points; 2 points each)

    a.

    b.

    c.

ESSAY: Answer the following questions using complete sentences.

38. Since reading Chapter 11 on questions and thinking of five sincere questions you have for God, record them here and explain why each is such an important question for you. (12 points)

39. Since setting up alone time with your Dad and/or Mom and asking them some of the questions from the textbook as well as some of your own, share how you feel that your communication with one or both of them could be improved. Include in your answer: (12 points)

    • 5 sample questions you could ask your parents to open up conversation.

    • 3 examples of when it would not be a good time to try to talk with your parent(s).

    • Why it is important to keep communication open with your parents.

    • What you have learned to improve your communication with your parents.

Total Health ································· Chapter 11 • Test Key

Unit 4: Spiritual Health   100 points

TRUE OR FALSE: Place a T for true or a F for false in front of the statements below concerning the place of questions in your life. (4 points; 1 points each)

1. __T__ Too many teens allow their minds to turn into non-thinking vegetables because they spend too much time in front of electronic media.
2. __F__ It's bad to ask questions because people don't like me if I do.
3. __T__ The human mind can be used to make inventions and discoveries—both good and bad.
4. __T__ It's okay to ask questions because that's the way that I develop my God-given thinking skills.

MATCHING (5 points; 1 points each): For each numbered item, place the letter of the correct answer in the space provided at the left of each item. Each answer can be used only once.

5. __C__ Martin Luther, church reformer

6. __E__ John Calvin, church reformer

7. __D__ John Wycliffe, church reformer, Bible translator

8. __B__ Charles Finney, cvangelist

9. __A__ John Wesley, founder of Methodism

A. What kind of method can we use to teach Christians to be holy and disciplined?

B. How can true revival be maintained?

C. Doesn't the Bible say that we are saved by faith and not by works?

D. Why can't I translate the Bible into the language of the common man?

E. How does the biblical doctrine of God's sovereignty apply to our daily lives?

LEADERS OR FOLLOWERS: Place L for leaders or F for followers in front of the following statements as to which they best describe. (12 points; 2 points each)

10. __L__ Ask good questions.
11. __L__ Control their TV and movie time.
12. __F__ Use most of their time "vegging out" with electronic entertainment.
13. __L__ Read interesting books.
14. __L__ Use their minds to think.
15. __F__ Aren't interested in reading, thinking or writing.

TRUE OR FALSE: (2 points; 1 point each) Place a C for "correctly used" or an I for "incorrectly used" in front of the following statements as they relate to the use of the word "comprehension".

16. __I__ Gary's car started to have problems due to a quick decrease in the comprehension in the engine.
17. __C__ When Katy listened to the preacher on the radio, she was not able to comprehend some of his points because he was using words that were too big for her.

TRUE OR FALSE: Place a T for true or a F for false in front of the following statements as they pertain to being good ways to develop the mind that God has given to you. (5 points; 1 point each)

18. __T__ Writing in a personal diary or journal.

19. __T__ Criticizing the TV shows and movies you watch.

20. __F__ Trying to reduce the amount of time you spending thinking upon what you're reading so that you can get through the book as fast as possible.

21. __T__ Doing your homework before you watch TV.

22. __T__ Riding your bike or talking to a friend instead of playing a computer game.

MATCHING: For each numbered item, place the letter of the correct answer in the space provided at the left of each item. Each answer can be used only once. (10 points; 2 points each)

23. __E__ Humility

24. __D__ Hypocrites

25. __A__ Countenance

26. __B__ Intellectual

27. __C__ Regress

A. Mental; having to do with your mind.

B. "Two-faced"; giving the impression that you have certain beliefs or feelings that you really don't have.

C. The expression on your face.

D. To go backwards.

E. Realizing your own limitations.

TRUE OR FALSE: Place a T for true or a F for false in front of each of the following statements as they relate to the subject of questions. (8 points; 2 points each)

28. __F__ There are not that many questions in the Bible.

29. __F__ God feels insecure and threatened whenever you ask Him a question.

30. __F__ God rejected people in the Scriptures whenever they asked Him a question.

31. __T__ Jesus used questions to cause people to think when He taught them.

SHORT ANSWER: Answer the following questions.

32. One of the foundations to all of your leadership skills is your reading and comprehension. List four things you can do in order to increase your reading skills. (8 points; 2 points each)

   a. *The next time you watch a movie, look at the credits and see what book the movie was taken from. Read the book upon which your favorite movie was based. Compare the book with the movie.*

   b. *Tell yourself that you're going to spend just as much time reading as you do watching TV or movies.*

   c. *Try not using any electronic entertainment for a day, a week, or more. See if you get better grades, develop more friendship, have fun learning something new, or get more good books read.*

   d. *Find a friend who likes to read the same kind of books that you do.*

   e. *Use a Bible translation that you really understand and like.*

   f. *Help to put together a home environment that is favorable to reading.*

33. What does it mean to allow your parents to "save face"? Why is this a sign of respect? (5 points)

One of the ways that you can show respect for your parents is in allowing them to "save face". As you mature, you're going to make some mistakes and so are your parents. Your parents have a lot of pressure on them to "be right" and "do right" most of the time. Because of this pressure, they usually won't appreciate it if you expose their mistakes in a direct or disrespectful way; some won't like it at all. But, as you get older, you're going to see legitimate problems in your parents. The fact is that everybody has weaknesses because we're all fallen and broken human beings.

34. If asking questions is good, when does it become wrong or bad? (4 points)

Questions are good as long as they come from a heart that is simply seeking the truth. An attitude of pride, trying to be obnoxious or trying to make someone be embarrassed or "Look bad" are ways that questioning can be wrong. Check your motives and the timing of when to ask what question.

35. Thinking biblically and asking intelligent questions are signs of the following three good, biblical qualities: (3 points)
    a. *knowledge*
    b. *wisdom*
    c. *humility*

36. What four books in the Bible are considered the Wisdom Books? (4 points)
    a. *Job*
    b. *Psalms*
    c. *Proverbs*
    d. *Ecclesiastes*

37. List three ways to show respect to your parent(s)—or to anyone. (6 points; 2 points each)
    a. *Look at them when they're talking to you.*
    b. *Acknowledge what they've said to you by repeating it back to them or saying, for example, "Yes, Mom."*
    c. *Ask them to reconsider by giving them a good reason if you are struggling with what they've just asked you to do.*
    d. *Saying "Please" more often.*
    e. *Showing a grateful spirit by saying "Thank you" more often.*

ESSAY: Answer the following questions using complete sentences.

38. Since reading Chapter 11 on questions and thinking of five sincere questions you have for God, record them here and explain why each is such an important question for you. (12 points)

    Answers may vary. E.g., Why did my parents get a divorce? Why am I so short? When can I think about dating? How do I know God's will for my life? Why do tragedies happen to Christians?

39. Since setting up alone time with your Dad and/or Mom and asking them some of the questions from the textbook as well as some of your own, share how you feel that your communication with one or both of them could be improved. Include in your answer: (12 points)

    - 5 sample questions you could ask your parents to open up conversation.
        - *What do you remember most clearly from when you were my age?*
        - *Were you a Christian when you were a teen?*
        - *How has God led you over the years?*
        - *What questions do you have to ask God?*
        - *How did God bring you and Mom/Dad together?*

    - 3 examples of when it would not be a good time to try to talk with your parent(s).
        - *when they're on the phone*
        - *when they're watching their favorite TV program or movie*
        - *when they're trying to meet a deadline*

    - Why it is important to keep communication open with your parents.
        - *to keep a good atmosphere in the home*
        - *to learn wise choices from them*
        - *to be accountable to them*

    - What you have learned to improve your communication with your parents.
        - *to show them respect*
        - *to ask them questions*
        - *to not be pushy*

196

Total Health ·········· **Chapter 12 • Quiz A**

Unit 4: Spiritual Health

Sections 12.1-12.2

15 Points

Name:_____

Date: _____

Score: _____

MATCHING: (2 points total; 1 point each) For each numbered item, place the letter of the correct answer in the space provided at the left of each item. Each answer can be used only once.

1. _____ Prayer
2. _____ Fear

A. A concern or anxiety about something real or imagined.

B. Talking to God and listening to hear what God would say to you.

SHORT ANSWER: Answer the following questions.

3. What 3 sources or factors have probably influenced your view of God the most? (3 points)

4. Explain how your parent's personality might affect the way you see God. (1 point)

5. What are two main goals of Bible reading or Bible meditation? (1 point; ½ point each)

6. What does it mean to "abide" in God throughout the day? (1 point)

TRUE OR FALSE: (6 points; 1 point each) Place a T for true or a F for false for each of the following statements as to whether they are accurate concerning your relationship with God.

7. _____ When you feel that praying isn't bringing you any closer to God, it could be that He is asking you to do something other than pray, e.g., go to your brother and tell him how you felt so upset when he eavesdropped on your telephone conversation the other day.

8. _____ When you feel that your prayers aren't being heard by God, it could never be that you have moral impurity or dishonesty in your life or are supposed to confront one of your friends about the same issue(s).

9. _____ Praying is like using your own inner hot-line to talk to God and listen to Him.

10. _____ God always answers your prayers right away. He never delays.

11. _____ If you're a Christian, you can "look within" to the Holy Spirit who lives inside of your heart and talk with Him anytime during the day.

12. _____ In order for God to listen to you when you pray, you should always pray like the person in your life who you view as the most spiritual.

MULTIPLE CHOICE: (1 point)

13. Place a check in the box for the one item below that is not a way that "helps" God hear us when we pray. Choose only one answer.
   ❑ When you are being yourself.
   ❑ When you are open about your needs and desires.
   ❑ When you are honest and sincere.
   ❑ When you command God to do something.
   ❑ When you leave the final results to Him.
   ❑ When you really want His glory.
   ❑ When you genuinely desire the good of someone else.

Total Health · Chapter 12 • Quiz A Key

Unit 4: Spiritual Health   15 points

Sections 12.1-12.2

MATCHING: (2 points total; 1 point each) For each numbered item, place the letter of the correct answer in the space provided at the left of each item. Each answer can be used only once.

1. __B__ Prayer

2. __A__ Fear

A. A concern or anxiety about something real or imagined.

B. Talking to God and listening to hear what God would say to you.

SHORT ANSWER: Answer the following questions.

3. What 3 sources or factors have probably influenced your view of God the most? (3 points)

   What your parents, teachers, and pastors have taught you about God is likely to be the same way that you think about Him.

4. Explain how your parent's personality might affect the way you see God. (1 point)

   If your parents are easy to talk to and very understanding, you'll probably see God in that way, too. But, if your parents are distant or too busy for you, you might begin to think that God is the same way—even though He isn't.

5. What are two main goals of Bible reading or Bible meditation? (1 point; 1/2 point each)

   To help you to love God more (develop a closer relationship with Him).

   To show you how to love people more like Jesus loves them.

6. What does it mean to "abide" in God throughout the day? (1 point)

   Keeping your prayer "hot-line" open to God all day. Talking to God, even briefly, throughout your day. Thanking Him as well as asking Him for guidance.

TRUE OR FALSE: (6 points; 1 point each) Place a T for true or a F for false for each of the following statements as to whether they are accurate concerning your relationship with God.

7. __T__ When you feel that praying isn't bringing you any closer to God, it could be that He is asking you to do something other than pray, e.g., go to your brother and tell him how you felt so upset when he eavesdropped on your telephone conversation the other day.

8. __F__ When you feel that your prayers aren't being heard by God, it could never be that you have moral impurity or dishonesty in your life or are supposed to confront one of your friends about the same issue(s).

9. __T__ Praying is like using your own inner hot-line to talk to God and listen to Him.

10. __F__ God always answers your prayers right away. He never delays.

11. __T__ If you're a Christian, you can "look within" to the Holy Spirit who lives inside of your heart and talk with Him anytime during the day.

12. __F__ In order for God to listen to you when you pray, you should always pray like the person in your life who you view as the most spiritual.

MULTIPLE CHOICE: (1 point)

13. Place a check in the box for the one item below that is not a way that "helps" God hear us when we pray. Choose only one answer.
    - ❏ When you are being yourself.
    - ❏ When you are open about your needs and desires.
    - ❏ When you are honest and sincere.
    - ☑ When you command God to do something.
    - ❏ When you leave the final results to Him.
    - ❏ When you really want His glory.
    - ❏ When you genuinely desire the good of someone else.

Total Health ·············· Chapter 12 • Quiz B

Unit 4: Spiritual Health

Sections 12.3-12.5

15 Points

Name:_____

Date: _____

Score: _____

SHORT ANSWER AND FILL IN THE BLANK: Answer the following questions.

1. "My life is like a _____ because God will have me take one step (piece) at a time." (1 point)

2. In the section, "What Are You Allowing to Influence Your Life?", what does the author say can be a very negative spiritual influence upon your life if you're not really careful? (2 points)

MULTIPLE CHOICE:

3. Place a check in the box of the *one* best definition of the word "destiny". (1 point)
   - ❑ Something special for you in your future.
   - ❑ A purpose that God has created for you.
   - ❑ A career or ministry that you've always wanted to do.
   - ❑ Marrying a good Christian.

4. From the options below, place a check in the box of the *one* best answer to the following question. What does the text say is the most important part of your divine destiny? (1 point)
   - ❑ Reaching as many people as possible for Christ.
   - ❑ Developing all of the spiritual gifts God has given to you.
   - ❑ Having a close, loving relationship with Jesus.
   - ❑ Being a missionary, if God would call you to the mission field.

5. Place a check in the box which contains the words which complete the following sentence from the very end of the textbook: "As it was with Adam and Eve, so it'll be in your life. Your future will be a giant unfolding of the results of all of your ____." (1 point)
   - ❑ Spiritual thoughts
   - ❑ Godly desires
   - ❑ Personal choices
   - ❑ Divine dreams

6. Place a check in the box of the one answer that best answers the following question: If your friends were having a negative effect upon your relationship with God, what do you think would probably be the best thing to do about it? (1 point)
   - ❑ Talk to my friends and try to get them to change their behavior.
   - ❑ Talk to my teachers about what they would suggest I should do.
   - ❑ Drop my old friends and get some new friends.

7. Place a check in the box of the one answer that best answers the following question: When you sin or make a mistake, how do you think God feels about you? (1 point)
   - ❏ He doesn't like me anymore.
   - ❏ He doesn't like my sin, but He still strongly loves me.
   - ❏ He loves me so much that He would never discipline me or cause me any pain.

8. The root reason why many teens are "pretenders" and "fake" their Christian faith is: (1 point)
   - ❏ They didn't make a commitment to Christ when they were children.
   - ❏ They're afraid and unwilling to pay the price of being a real Christian.
   - ❏ They don't have strong Christian parents.

9. Place a check in the box for every answer listed below from the student text which answers the following question: What are some major hindrances to you fulfilling your divine destiny? (3 points)
   - ❏ When you don't feel good about how God made you.
   - ❏ When you make a mistake, get into trouble, and feel that God would never use you.
   - ❏ When your family is a non-Christian family.
   - ❏ When you don't know all that your future holds.

TRUE OR FALSE: Place a T for true or a F for false for each of the following statements as to whether they help to answer the question, "How is your life like a puzzle?" (3 points)

10. _____ My life is like a puzzle because God will have me take one step (piece) at a time.

11. _____ My life is like a puzzle because God will show me a picture of my whole life ahead of time, just like the photos of completed puzzles on jigsaw puzzle boxes.

12. _____ My life is like a puzzle because if I don't know what is the next piece to fit into it, all I have to do is to ask God, and He will show me.

Total Health • **Chapter 12 • Quiz B Key**

Unit 4: Spiritual Health   15 points

Sections 12.3-12.5

SHORT ANSWER AND FILL IN THE BLANK: Answer the following questions.

1. "My life is like a _____*puzzle*_____ because God will have me take one step (piece) at a time." (1 point)

2. In the section, "What Are You Allowing to Influence Your Life?", what does the author say can be a very negative spiritual influence upon your life if you're not really careful? (2 points)
   the wrong kind of friends

MULTIPLE CHOICE:

3. Place a check in the box of the *one* best definition of the word "destiny". (1 point)
   - ❏ Something special for you in your future.
   - ☑ A purpose that God has created for you.
   - ❏ A career or ministry that you've always wanted to do.
   - ❏ Marrying a good Christian.

4. From the options below, place a check in the box of the *one* best answer to the following question. What does the text say is the most important part of your divine destiny? (1 point)
   - ❏ Reaching as many people as possible for Christ.
   - ❏ Developing all of the spiritual gifts God has given to you.
   - ☑ Having a close, loving relationship with Jesus.
   - ❏ Being a missionary, if God would call you to the mission field.

5. Place a check in the box which contains the words which complete the following sentence from the very end of the textbook: "As it was with Adam and Eve, so it'll be in your life. Your future will be a giant unfolding of the results of all of your ____." (1 point)
   - ❏ Spiritual thoughts
   - ❏ Godly desires
   - ☑ Personal choices
   - ❏ Divine dreams

6. Place a check in the box of the one answer that best answers the following question: If your friends were having a negative effect upon your relationship with God, what do you think would probably be the best thing to do about it? (1 point)
   - ❏ Talk to my friends and try to get them to change their behavior.
   - ❏ Talk to my teachers about what they would suggest I should do.
   - ☑ Drop my old friends and get some new friends.

7. Place a check in the box of the one answer that best answers the following question: When you sin or make a mistake, how do you think God feels about you? (1 point)

    ❏ He doesn't like me anymore.

    ☑ He doesn't like my sin, but He still strongly loves me.

    ❏ He loves me so much that He would never discipline me or cause me any pain.

8. The root reason why many teens are "pretenders" and "fake" their Christian faith is: (1 point)

    ❏ They didn't make a commitment to Christ when they were children.

    ☑ They're afraid and unwilling to pay the price of being a real Christian.

    ❏ They don't have strong Christian parents.

9. Place a check in the box for every answer listed below from the student text which answers the following question: What are some major hindrances to you fulfilling your divine destiny? (3 points)

    ☑ When you don't feel good about how God made you.

    ☑ When you make a mistake, get into trouble, and feel that God would never use you.

    ❏ When your family is a non-Christian family.

    ☑ When you don't know all that your future holds.

TRUE OR FALSE: Place a T for true or a F for false for each of the following statements as to whether they help to answer the question, "How is your life like a puzzle?" (3 points)

10. _T_ My life is like a puzzle because God will have me take one step (piece) at a time.

11. _F_ My life is like a puzzle because God will show me a picture of my whole life ahead of time, just like the photos of completed puzzles on jigsaw puzzle boxes.

12. _T_ My life is like a puzzle because if I don't know what is the next piece to fit into it, all I have to do is to ask God, and He will show me.

Total Health ·································· **Chapter 12 • Test**

Unit 4: Spiritual Health

100 Points

Name:_____

Date: _____

Score: _____

TRUE AND FALSE: Place a T for true or a F for false for each of the following statements as to whether they are accurate concerning your relationship with God. (12 points; 2 points each)

1. _____ When you feel that praying isn't bringing you any closer to God, it could be that He is asking you to do something other than pray, e.g, go to your brother and tell him how you felt so upset when he eavesdropped on your telephone conversation the other day.

2. _____ When you feel that your prays aren't being heard by God, it could never be that you have moral impurity or dishonesty in your life or are supposed to confront one of your friends about the same issue(s).

3. _____ Praying is like using your own inner hot-line to talk to God and listen to Him.

4. _____ God always answers your prayers right away. He never delays.

5. _____ If you're a Christian, you can "look within" to the Holy Spirit who lives inside of your heart and talk with Him anytime during the day.

6. _____ In order for God to listen to you when you pray, you should always pray like the person in your life who you view as the most spiritual.

7. For each numbered definition below, place either P for prayer or F for fear in the space provided. (14 points; 2 points each)

(1)_____ An anxiety about something real.

(2)_____ Talking to God.

(3)_____ A concern about something imagined.

(4)_____ Listening to hear what God would say to you.

(5)_____ Asking Jesus to help your friends.

(6)_____ An emotion that the devil likes to stir up in teens.

(7)_____ A feeling that can sometimes help you to be safe.

MULTIPLE CHOICE: For the following questions, place a check in the box of the most appropriate answer(s).

8. What is the *one* item below that is *not* a way that "helps" God hear us when we pray. Choose only one answer. (3 points)

❑ When you are being yourself.

❑ When you are open about your needs and desires.

❑ When you are honest and sincere.

❑ When you command God to do something by faith.

❑ When you leave the final results to Him.

❑ When you sincerely want all the glory to go to God.

❑ When you genuinely desire the good of someone else.

9. From the options below, what is the *one* best definition of the word "destiny". (3 points)
    ❑ Something special for you in your future.
    ❑ A purpose that God has created you for.
    ❑ A career or ministry that you've always wanted to do.
    ❑ Marrying a good Christian.

10. What does the text say is *the most* important part of your divine destiny? (3 points)
    ❑ Reaching as many people as possible for Christ.
    ❑ Developing all of the spiritual gifts God has given to you.
    ❑ Having a close, loving relationship with Jesus.
    ❑ Being a missionary, if God would call you to the mission field.

11. When you sin or make a mistake, how do you think God feels about you? (one answer; 3 points)
    ❑ He doesn't like me anymore.
    ❑ He doesn't like my sin, but He still strongly loves me.
    ❑ He loves me so much that He would never discipline me or cause me any pain.

12. The root reason why many teens are "pretenders" and "fake" their Christian faith is: (one answer; 3 points)
    ❑ They didn't make a commitment to Christ when they were children.
    ❑ They're afraid and unwilling to pay the price of being a real Christian.
    ❑ They don't have strong Christian parents.

13. What are some major hindrances in you fulfilling your divine destiny? (more than one answer; 6 points; 3 points each)
    ❑ When you don't feel good about how God made you.
    ❑ When you make a mistake, get into trouble, and feel that God would never use you.
    ❑ When your family is a non-Christian family.
    ❑ When you don't know all that your future holds.

14. If your friends were having a negative effect upon your relationship with God, what do you think would probably be the one best thing to do about it? (2 points)
    ❑ Talk to your friends and try to get them to change their behavior.
    ❑ Talk to your teachers what they would suggest I should do.
    ❑ Drop your old friends and get some new friends.

TRUE OR FALSE: Place a T for true or a F for false for each of the following statements as to whether they help to answer the question, "How is your life like a puzzle?" (3 points; 1 point each)

15. _____ My life is like a puzzle because God will have me take one step (piece) at a time.

16. _____ My life is like a puzzle because God will show me a picture of my whole life ahead of time, just like the photos of completed puzzles on jigsaw puzzle boxes.

17. _____ My life is like a puzzle because if I don't know what is the next piece to fit into it, all I have to do is to ask God and He will show me.

206

SHORT ANSWER AND FILL IN THE BLANK: Answer the following questions.

18. "As it was with Adam and Eve, so it'll be in your life. Your future will be a giant unfolding of the results of all of your _____." (4 points)
    A. Spiritual thoughts
    B. Godly desires
    C. Personal choices
    D. Divine dreams

19. Explain how your parents' personality might affect the way you see God. (3 points)

20. What does it mean to "abide" in God throughout the day? (3 points)

21. What are two main goals of Bible reading or Bible meditation? (4 points; 2 points each)
    a.

    b.

22. What 3 sources or factors have probably influenced your view of God the most? (6 points; 2 points each)

23. In the section, "What Are You Allowing to Influence Your Life?", what does the author say can be a very negative spiritual influence upon your life if you're not really careful? (2 points)

24. You can learn to hear God's voice—personally. List five ways of how God might speak to you. (5 points)
    a.

    b.

    c.

    d.

    e.

207

ESSAY: Answer the following questions using complete sentences.

25. What does it mean for a teenager to "count the cost" of being a Christian? Include in your answer:

   • What does it mean to "fake" your Christianity? (5 points)

   • Why might teens "fake" their Christianity? (5 points)

   • How do you think "faking" makes God feel? (5 points)

26. The Bible says that Satan is the "father of lies" in John 8:44. How might knowing this help you to recognize his schemes against you? (10 points)

Total Health • Chapter 12 • Test Key

Unit 4: Spiritual Health   100 points

TRUE AND FALSE: Place a T for true or a F for false for each of the following statements as to whether they are accurate concerning your relationship with God. (12 points; 2 points each)

1. _T_ When you feel that praying isn't bringing you any closer to God, it could be that He is asking you to do something other than pray, e.g, go to your brother and tell him how you felt so upset when he eavesdropped on your telephone conversation the other day.

2. _F_ When you feel that your prays aren't being heard by God, it could never be that you have moral impurity or dishonesty in your life or are supposed to confront one of your friends about the same issue(s).

3. _T_ Praying is like using your own inner hot-line to talk to God and listen to Him.

4. _F_ God always answers your prayers right away. He never delays.

5. _T_ If you're a Christian, you can "look within" to the Holy Spirit who lives inside of your heart and talk with Him anytime during the day.

6. _F_ In order for God to listen to you when you pray, you should always pray like the person in your life who you view as the most spiritual.

7. For each numbered definition below, place either P for prayer or F for fear in the space provided. (14 points; 2 points each)

(1)_F_ An anxiety about something real.

(2)_P_ Talking to God.

(3)_F_ A concern about something imagined.

(4)_P_ Listening to hear what God would say to you.

(5)_P_ Asking Jesus to help your friends.

(6)_F_ An emotion that the devil likes to stir up in teens.

(7)_F_ A feeling that can sometimes help you to be safe.

MULTIPLE CHOICE: For the following questions, place a check in the box of the most appropriate answer(s).

8. What is the *one* item below that is *not* a way that "helps" God hear us when we pray. Choose only one answer. (3 points)
   ❑ When you are being yourself.
   ❑ When you are open about your needs and desires.
   ❑ When you are honest and sincere.
   ☑ When you command God to do something by faith.
   ❑ When you leave the final results to Him.
   ❑ When you sincerely want all the glory to go to God.
   ❑ When you genuinely desire the good of someone else.

209

9. From the options below, what is the *one* best definition of the word "destiny". (3 points)
   - ❑ Something special for you in your future.
   - ☑ A purpose that God has created you for.
   - ❑ A career or ministry that you've always wanted to do.
   - ❑ Marrying a good Christian.

10. What does the text say is *the most* important part of your divine destiny? (3 points)
   - ❑ Reaching as many people as possible for Christ.
   - ❑ Developing all of the spiritual gifts God has given to you.
   - ☑ Having a close, loving relationship with Jesus.
   - ❑ Being a missionary, if God would call you to the mission field.

11. When you sin or make a mistake, how do you think God feels about you? (one answer; 3 points)
   - ❑ He doesn't like me anymore.
   - ☑ He doesn't like my sin, but He still strongly loves me.
   - ❑ He loves me so much that He would never discipline me or cause me any pain.

12. The root reason why many teens are "pretenders" and "fake" their Christian faith is: (one answer; 3 points)
   - ❑ They didn't make a commitment to Christ when they were children.
   - ☑ They're afraid and unwilling to pay the price of being a real Christian.
   - ❑ They don't have strong Christian parents.

13. What are some major hindrances in you fulfilling your divine destiny? (more than one answer; 6 points; 3 points each)
   - ☑ When you don't feel good about how God made you.
   - ☑ When you make a mistake, get into trouble, and feel that God would never use you.
   - ❑ When your family is a non-Christian family.
   - ❑ When you don't know all that your future holds.

14. If your friends were having a negative effect upon your relationship with God, what do you think would probably be the one best thing to do about it? (2 points)
   - ❑ Talk to your friends and try to get them to change their behavior.
   - ❑ Talk to your teachers what they would suggest I should do.
   - ☑ Drop your old friends and get some new friends.

TRUE OR FALSE: Place a T for true or a F for false for each of the following statements as to whether they help to answer the question, "How is your life like a puzzle?" (3 points; 1 point each)

15. __T__ My life is like a puzzle because God will have me take one step (piece) at a time.

16. __F__ My life is like a puzzle because God will show me a picture of my whole life ahead of time, just like the photos of completed puzzles on jigsaw puzzle boxes.

17. __T__ My life is like a puzzle because if I don't know what is the next piece to fit into it, all I have to do is to ask God and He will show me.

SHORT ANSWER AND FILL IN THE BLANK: Answer the following questions.

18. "As it was with Adam and Eve, so it'll be in your life. Your future will be a giant unfolding of the results of all of your _____*personal choices*_____." (4 points)

    A. Spiritual thoughts

    B. Godly desires

    C. Personal choices

    D. Divine dreams

19. Explain how your parents' personality might affect the way you see God. (3 points)

    If your parents are easy to talk to and very understanding, you'll probably see God in that way, too. But, if your parents are distant or too busy for you, you might begin to think that God is the say way—even though He isn't.

20. What does it mean to "abide" in God throughout the day? (3 points)

    Keeping your prayer "hot-line" open to God all day. Talking to God, even briefly, throughout your day. Thanking Him as well as asking Him for guidance.

21. What are two main goals of Bible reading or Bible meditation? (4 points; 2 points each)

    a. To help you to love God more (develop a closer relationship with Him)

    b. To show you how to love people more like Jesus loves them.

22. What 3 sources or factors have probably influenced your view of God the most? (6 points; 2 points each)

    What your parents, teachers, and pastors have taught you about God is likely to be the same way that you think about Him.

23. In the section, "What Are You Allowing to Influence Your Life?", what does the author say can be a very negative spiritual influence upon your life if you're not really careful? (2 points)

    The wrong kind of friends

24. You can learn to hear God's voice—personally. List five ways of how God might speak to you. (5 points)

    a. Through the Bible

    b. Through prayer

    c. Through other Christians

    d. Through the Holy Spirit

    e. Through giving us strong convictions,

    ALSO: worship, conscience, dreams, whispers in your heart, thoughts in your mind, circum-stances and experiences.

ESSAY: Answer the following questions using complete sentences.

25. What does it mean for a teenager to "count the cost" of being a Christian? Include in your answer:

  • What does it mean to "fake" your Christianity? (5 points)

  • Why might teens "fake" their Christianity? (5 points)

  • How do you think "faking" makes God feel? (5 points)

  · *To "count the cost" of being a Christian means that teenagers need to come to Christ not just for all of the good, positive things that they feel that He will give to them. But, they need to come follow Jesus also knowing that Christ is going to change their lives and allow them to be rejected and criticized for their beliefs.*

  · *It means that teenagers pretend to be Christians with impure motives.*

  · *They may want others to accept them, they may be interested in a "cute" Christian guy or girl, they may be afraid of disappointing their parents, etc, but they are not sincere or genuine in what they outwardly do for the Lord.*

  · *This makes God feel sad and sick because He wants all teens to have a real relationship with Him.*

26. The Bible says that Satan is the "father of lies" in John 8:44. How might knowing this help you to recognize his schemes against you? (10 points)

  Answers will vary. They will probably include believing and obeying the Scriptures rather than friends who may be a negative influence over your life because they may encourage you to drink, smoke, have sex, steal, lie, yell at parents, cuss God out, watch impure movies, gossip, etc.

Student Text Chapter Review Answer Keys

Chapter 1 Review Answers

Defining the Terms

(If the following terms are not clearly defined in this chapter, use the definition from a dictionary.)

Temptation: something that allures or draws someone especially to evil

Consequences: the effect, outcome or result of something

Influence: the power of persons or things to produce effects on others

Habit: a pattern of behavior established from repetition

Deception: the act of misleading by false appearance or statement, to trick

Soul: a person's mind, will, and emotions

Total Health: physical, mental, social and spiritual well-being

Recalling the Facts

1. Satan began to question Eve about what God really had said. He wanted to isolate her from Adam and from God. He tried to trick her by lying to her about God's intentions. He brought doubt into her mind.

2. Their eyes were opened to good and evil. They recognized they were naked. Deception brought fear and separation from God. Adam and Eve hid from God and felt afraid of God. They did not feel they could tell Him what they had done.

3. Adam and Eve's "forbidden fruit" was the tree in the middle of the garden. It was God's commandment to them not to eat from it. To us, it's something that God wants us to stay away from.

4. The Tree of Life means to be dependent upon God, knowing your need for others, to be involved, talking with safe adults, telling the truth and being open and transparent about your thoughts and feelings. The Tree of Death leads you to be independent from God, seeing no need for others, being isolated, not talking with safe adults, covering up, being dishonest and being closed and afraid to share thoughts and feelings.

5. God called for them and sought them out.

6. Physically: disease, decay, death, and pain in childbirth. Adam would have to work hard in manual labor and struggle for food.

Mentally: Mankind would struggle with the animals. Experience mental and emotional stress from fear of bad climate and dangerous beasts.

Socially: Severe conflict between human beings. Jealousy, hatred, violence.

Spiritually: The spirit of mankind, which was once in close union with God, would now be separated because of sin. Feelings of loneliness and isolation.

Applying the Truth

1. Do not be wise in your own eyes, don't be influenced by others or "go along" with an evil crowd of people who would want you to do wrong. Flee evil, don't hang around just to "check things out".

2. Pressure to disobey your parents, temptation to give into peer pressure of immorality, gossip, drinking alcohol, trying drugs and tobacco. A desire to do things that you know will not be pleasing to God.

3. Personal reflection; the answer is subjective. Encourage discussion of the importance of talking to a safe, Christian adult they can trust. Positive choice: a person who wants them to please the Lord, the Bible, and their parents. Negative choice: a person who does not care about what is right or wrong; does not support them by praying for or with them; is not a strong, growing Christian.

4. Possible answers may include: choice of friends, study habits in school, food choices, decision to try tobacco, drugs, or alcohol, decision to get involved with the opposite sex, the decision to improve their communication with their parent(s).

Chapter 2 Review Answers

Defining the Terms

Healthy: a state of physical, mental, social and spiritual well-being

Cells: the basic building blocks of the body from which all larger parts are formed

Tissues: similar cells organized into specialized groups to carry out particular functions

Arteriosclerosis: hardening of the arteries

Organ: two or more tissues grouped together to perform a singular function

Arteries: carry oxygenated blood away from the heart

Veins: carry blood that lacks oxygen (deoxygenated blood) back to the heart

Capillaries: the smallest blood vessels

Plasma: the liquid portion of the blood

Red blood cells: the portion of the blood that carries oxygen

White blood cells: the portion of the blood that fights germs, viruses, and diseases

Platelets: the portion of the blood that helps the blood to clot

Blood pressure: the force that your blood puts on the inside walls of your blood vessels

Stroke: when the flow of blood to one part of the brain is severely restricted or cut off

Pharynx: the throat

Trachea: carries air to the lungs

Esophagus: a passageway that carries food to the stomach

Epiglottis: a small flap of skin that prevents food from entering the trachea

Lungs: large, soft cone-shaped organs used for breathing

Diaphragm: a large muscle that separates the chest from the abdomen

Skeletal muscles: muscles that cause the body to move

Smooth muscles: muscles found in the digestive system and blood vessels which provide movement within the body

Cardiac muscle: the heart muscle

Digestion: the process by which food is broken down and made useful for the body

Alimentary canal: a long muscular tube that extends from the mouth to the anus

Large intestine: the cecum, colon, rectum, and anal canal; moves waste through the body

Small intestine: where most of the digestion and absorption of nutrients occurs

Kidneys: two bean-shaped organs that cleanse the blood of impurities and send it back to the bloodstream

Homeostasis: a balanced, stable internal environment inside the body

Hormones: chemicals released by the glands of the endocrine system; often called "chemical messengers"

Pituitary gland: located in the brain, the master gland releasing the growth hormone

Thyroid gland: hormones released from the thyroid control how fast the body metabolizes (uses) food for energy

Adrenal glands: release hormones in response to certain types of stress; responsible for the "fight-or-flight" response

Ovaries: the glands of the female reproductive system, located inside the female body; gradually release hormones responsible for female sex characteristics

Testes: the glands of the male reproductive system, located outside the male body; gradually release hormones responsible for male sex characteristics

Recalling the Facts

1. Each individual cell is living, moving, sensing, breathing, reproducing, growing, eliminating, eating/drinking.

2. Epithelial tissues: cover all body surfaces inside and out

   Connective tissues: bind structures together providing support and protection

   Muscle tissues: provide movement

   Nerve tissues: receive and transmit impulses to various parts of the body

3. The circulatory system is like a major transportation system. It transports fuel to the body, carries wastes to the liver and kidneys, sends cells to fight disease, and transports hormones throughout the body.

4. You can choose to hold your breath, but sooner or later your body's need for oxygen will overcome your own ability to resist, and you will gasp for air.

5. Support, protection, manufacture, storage

6. Skeletal muscles work in pairs. While one muscle contracts (shortens) the other extends (lengthens). A baseball player swings a bat (triceps and biceps muscles). Another pair would be the quad and the hamstring of the thigh, or the back and stomach muscles.

7. The purpose of the excretory system is to provide ways for waste to be removed from the body. Even if a car owner tuned his engine and put fresh oil into it daily, if the exhaust system was not working, there would be something wrong with the car. What would happen to your car if you put a potato in the exhaust pipe? Liken this to constipation!

Applying the Truth

1. Helped: All systems are helped in some way, but the circulatory, cardiovascular, respiratory, muscular, skeletal, digestive and excretory systems are most directly affected. More efficient use of oxygen, strengthens the heart muscle, increases oxygen to the blood, strengthens the bones and muscles for protection and longevity, improves digestion and absorption of nutrients, and improves the ability of the elimination of wastes.

2. Every body system is hurt by poor nutrition; however, the circulatory, cardiovascular, digestive, and excretory systems are more directly affected. Poor diet causes hardening of the arteries, lowers ability to fight off diseases, makes the heart work harder than normal, slows down the digestive system, and makes the excretory system become less efficient. Teens should consider less junk food that is high in salt, fat and sugar. Diet soda pop with its dangerous chemicals as well as regular soda pop that is high in sugar, should be limited in their diets. Eat

more fresh vegetables and fruit to help these systems.

3. • The vomiting reflex: saves us from poisons

• Fertilization of a single cell

• The miles of nerves that run through the body

• The incredible numbers of blood cells constantly flowing through the body

• The body's ability to maintain a balanced internal environment despite the outside temperature, stress, etc.

• The difference between the male and female bone structure for a specific purpose: the female pelvis created for delivery of children

Chapter 3 Review Answers

Defining the Terms

Balanced diet: making food choices that include a wide variety from all that God has given to us in nature

Calorie: a unit of heat that your body uses for activity

Empty calories: those foods that don't have any nutritive value

Nutrients: substances in foods that your body needs (proteins, carbohydrates, fats, vitamins, minerals and water)

Proteins: a string of amino acids used by the body to build new cells and tissues

Essential amino acids: eight amino acids that your body does not produce naturally and must get from the foods you eat

Vegetarian diet: a diet that typically excludes animal products

Carbohydrates: Sugars and starches that the body uses for energy

Fats: concentrated sources of energy that can provide twice as much energy than carbohydrates

Saturated fat: these fats are solid at room temperature which tend to increase blood cholesterol

Cholesterol: a fatty substance in the blood which increases the risk of heart disease

Unsaturated fats: usually liquid at room temperature and don't tend to raise blood cholesterol

Vitamins: organic substances the body needs in small amounts

RDA: Recommended Daily Allowance

Water-soluble: vitamins that dissolve in water and can pass through the body

Fat-soluble: vitamins that don't dissolve in water and can be stored in the body

Minerals: inorganic substances that are essential for the body

Metabolic rate: the speed at which your body burns calories

Diet: all the foods you choose to eat on a regular basis

Overweight: weighing more than the desired weight for age, sex, height and frame size

Obese: weighing more than 20% over one's ideal weight

Anorexia: self-induced starvation

Bulimia: a pattern of "binging" and "purging"

Chronic overeating: the habit of eating more food than your body needs

Recalling the Facts

1. The Food Pyramid recommends 6-11 servings of whole grains and high-fiber foods. Next, 2-4 servings of fruit and 3-5 of vegetables. The dairy section suggests 2-3 servings and the protein group 2-3 as well. Fats and sugars should be minimal. If I were to adjust the Food Pyramid, I would have the base category be filled with fresh fruits and vegetables and then the next group be the whole grains.

2. Saturated fats are solid at room temperature and tend to raise blood cholesterol. Unsaturated fats are liquid at room temperature and do not tend to raise blood cholesterol. Saturated fats are the most dangerous because they increase the chance of heart disease and other diseases. Butter is a saturated fat and vegetable oil is an unsaturated fat.

3. Water is the most common nutrient in your body. Without water, you would die. Your body uses water for cleansing of waste and toxins, lubricating joints, transporting nutrients, regulating body temperature, losing weight, and digesting food.

4. A food journal shows eating patterns. How much and what kind of food you eat at various times of the day. Sometimes you may eat and not know why or remember how much ("How many cookies did I just eat?"). You can make changes in your diet after evaluating "weak" times during the day when you may have the tendency to overeat or eat the wrong kinds of food.

5. Answers may vary, but some ideas include: Eat less sugar and sodium, drink more water, increase dietary fiber, try to maintain ideal weight without doing fad diets, eat a variety of foods and eat less saturated fat.

6. Fad diets are dangerous because usually they make promises that are unhealthy for your body. Many diet drinks have tons of sugar and lack the vital nutrients necessary to keep your body functioning (for example, enough fiber for regular bowel movements). Going on a diet makes you think of the short-term because it is an "on" and "off" decision rather than a lifestyle change.

Applying the Truth

1. A pizza contains carbohydrates, vegetables, and protein. A healthy pizza order would include low-fat cheeses and a whole-wheat crust, topped with lots of vegetables.

2. Keys to a great food journal are: (1) Be honest and write down everything I eat. (2) Be exact in writing down what I eat. (3) Be accountable to someone. (4) Fill in the comment section to help me understand why and when I eat certain foods. These will be hard because I must take extra time actually to think about what I am eating and how much. Then I have to be honest and share my food choices with another person—this can be embarrassing, especially if I don't choose the right person.

3. Answers may vary based on a person's previous knowledge of the Food Pyramid. Some answers may include: the number of servings for the bread, cereal group, or the fact that fruits and vegetables were not on the bottom. Each student may make dietary changes under the Food Pyramid based on their current eating habits.

4. Package labeling can be misleading because: the fancy packaging, the claims for being "fat-free" or "lite". Serving sizes can be misleading because they may be unusually small for the food product. Labels may also leave out specific amounts of ingredients such as hydrogenated oils and tropical oils.

5. Imagine you have a friend who seems to have poor eating habits and you are very concerned. How might you determine if they have a problem with anorexia or bulimia?

What might you say and/or do to help your friend?

Watch your friend closely for signs of self-starvation, over-exercising, using the bathroom after meals (vomiting or purging), or an extreme concern about watching her weight. If you have a good relationship with the individual and his/her family, you could try to talk with the parent(s) about your concern without her knowing. Ask her if she feels she is having a problem and wants your support and help. Do not criticize or tease her about her body or eating habits. Suggest a good book for you or your friend to read such as: *Walking the Thin Line: Anorexia and Bulimia, the Battle Can Be Won* by Pam Vredevelt; *The Monster Within: Overcoming Bulimia*; *The Courage to Go On*; or *Food for the Hungry Heart* by Cynthia Rowland McClure.

Chapter 4 Review Answers

Defining the Terms

Fitness: the ability of your mind and body to work together to their highest possible level

Cardiovascular fitness: the condition of the heart

Atrophy: occurs when a long period of time lapses between workouts and the muscles decrease in size and strength

Aerobic: when your muscles demand more oxygen than normal during an activity

Anaerobic: short bursts of activity without the use of much oxygen

Muscular fitness: the measurement of your muscle strength and muscle endurance

Flexibility: the ability to move your joints and muscles through a full range of motion

Body composition: the relationship between your fat and lean (muscle) body weight

Lifetime sports: activities that a person can participate in throughout a lifetime

Recalling the Facts

1. List of 16 is on page 70 of student text.

2. Without strong heart, lungs, and blood vessels working together to supply oxygenated blood to the whole body, without strong cardiovascular fitness, it would not matter how much weight you could lift if you died from a heart attack!

3. Aerobic exercise is activity that requires oxygen to perform. Swimming, running, and playing basketball are examples of aerobic exercise. It is important to include aerobic exercise in your life because it improves your cardiovascular fitness. Anaerobic exercise is activity that does not require much oxygen to perform. Anaerobic exercise is important for muscular strength and coordination development. Weightlifting, sprinting, and golf are examples of anaerobic activity.

4. A person should listen to his/her body because pain is the signal that something is wrong. There may be slight pain in stretching or exercising but you should never push past the point of pain. The nerve reflex protects your muscle by sending the pain signal. When you stretch too far, you are tightening the very muscles you are trying to loosen.

5. The warm-up prepares your muscles for activity. The body temperature must rise enough to increase the body temperature. Stretching should occur after the body is warm. A warm-down is important because the muscles need to re-

lease the build-up of lactic acid from the workout, and will decrease the muscle soreness, cramping, nausea or lightheadedness that can occur after a workout. Both a proper warm-up and warmdown help prevent injuries.

Applying the Truth

1. Regular aerobic exercise helps control a person's weight because of the extra calories that are burned through activity. Increase in muscle mass also helps because muscles burn more calories than fat. Teenagers can increase their exercise by joining an athletic team, riding their bike to school or other locations, getting involved with yard work or playing a non-competitive sport with friends.

2. An accidental workout means to increase your activity level when you don't even know you are doing it. It is making exercise and movement a fun and enjoyable part of your daily life, e.g., riding horses, bike riding, skateboarding, jumping rope, etc.

3. Comparing with your peers concerning appearance and skill. Comparing is one of the greatest enemies to your mind because it will either make you feel superior to others who aren't as good as you, or make you feel inferior to others who are better than you. God never intended for you to compare yourself with others. God only expects you to do your best and become the finest person you can become with the resources He's given to you.

Chapter 5 Review Answers

Defining the Terms

Homeostasis: a balanced, stable internal environment in the body

Disease: any condition that negatively affects the healthy and normal functioning of your mind or body

Infectious disease: caused by germs that spread from one person to another

Noninfectious disease: caused by heredity, the environment, and/or a person's lifestyle

Germs or Pathogens: tiny particles that may be plant or animal that cause disease

Symptoms: reactions from your body (stuffy nose, sore throat), that indicate that it is trying to fight an intruder or infection. Your body redirects its energy to fight the germ.

Viruses: smaller than bacteria and attack individual cells. They are responsible for the common cold, chicken pox, measles, and AIDS.

Bacteria: single-celled tiny organisms that attack your body. Strep throat, pneumonia, and some STDs are caused by bacteria.

Resident bacteria: "friendly" bacteria that your body needs

Antibodies: protein molecules produced by your white blood cells to fight off germs

Lymphocytes: white blood cells that fight off germs

Vaccine: weakened or destroyed cells of a particular germ that are injected into a person to produce enough antibodies to keep a person from contracting the disease

STD: sexually transmitted disease(s) (venereal disease) that pass from one person to another through sexual contact

Conviction(s): a person's strong belief on a particular issue

AIDS: Acquired Immunodeficiency Syndrome

HIV: Human Immunodeficiency Virus

Cancer: a disease which occurs when abnormal cells grow out of control

Tumor: masses of abnormal cells

Carcinogen: any natural or man-made substance that tends to produce cancer

Congenital: occurring at birth

Insulin: a hormone produced by the pancreas to control how the body uses sugar

Diabetes type I: insulin-dependent where the pancreas produces little or no insulin

Diabetes type II: non-insulin dependent where the pancreas does not produce enough insulin to meet the body's needs or the body can't use it correctly

Recalling the Facts

1. The body works very hard to maintain a stable and balanced internal environment so that each system functions efficiently for maximum health.

2. Germs can be spread in four ways: contact with an airborne germ, contact with an infected person, contact with infected animals, and contact with objects that an infected person has handled. From the time you become infected to the time you develop symptoms is called the incubation period, during which you are highly contagious.

3. Your body has both good (resident) bacteria and bad (illness-causing) bacteria. The body needs good bacteria to fight off the germs that invade it. Antibiotics kill both the good and bad bacteria, so you need to replace the good bacteria in your body.

4. Most germs are carried through contact with an infected person or infected item. Keeping your hands washed is the best form of defense against germs.

5. The skin is the first line of defense. The mucous membranes in your mouth, nose, and throat protect you from invading germs. The hairs in-

side your nose help keep small particles out. If germs have invaded your body, your white blood cells begin to produce special proteins called antibodies to fight them. When an individual cell is invaded by a germ, the body produces interferon to inform the other cells to fight the germ. If the virus cannot enter the other cells, then the infection has been stopped. A fever also works to burn off an invader.

6. Sexual abstinence

7. • Genetic make-up (heredity)
   • Lifestyle habits
   • Environmental factors
   • Occupational hazards
   • Your body's reaction to a virus

A person can directly control lifestyle, some elements of the environment, and their occupational choice. Heredity and your body's reaction to a virus (that is if you are keeping yourself as healthy as possible) are out of your direct control.

8. • Discover if you have any heart disease in your family.
   • Have a healthy lifestyle that includes a diet of fresh fruits and vegetables, and limit the fats and salt.
   • Exercise regularly to keep your heart fit and to decrease the effects of stress.

Applying the Truth

1. Even though Kristen was young when she got sick, she had a normal reaction to such bad news. Her attitude about living life to its fullest was positive even in the worst circumstances. God is sovereign in all His ways even though we don't always understand why things happen.

2. "Listen to your body" means to pay special attention to the symptoms you feel and your changing health. Maybe certain foods upset your stomach or you don't do well when you do not get enough sleep. You can change some health habits as you learn to listen to your body.

3. The Word of God, faith in God's power, faith in God's control

4. Lifestyle includes: food choices (consumption of alcohol, drugs, coffee, soda pop, processed foods), amount of exercise, involvement with the opposite sex.

5. It is important to know what you believe and why you believe it before you find yourself in a compromising situation. Often people do things they will regret because they have not developed strong convictions before a temptation faces them.

Chapter 6 Review Answers

Defining the Terms

Mature: showing good development and growth: physically, mentally, emotionally, socially and spiritually

Confident: no feelings of inferiority

Personal identity: to know who you are in Christ

Jealousy: feeling of resentment against another for having a success or talent that you want to have

Pride: to think yourself better than you really are; an "I don't need anyone"/"I'm better than others" attitude

Character: what you are on the inside, what you do when no one is watching

Self-esteem: the way you feel about yourself

Recalling the Facts

1. • *Physical:* possible acne, increase in height and weight, needing to shower more often
   • *Mental (emotional):* increased stress, feelings of independence, inability to "relate" to adults, and that general feeling that "no one understands"
   • *Social:* possible increased tension at home, attraction to the opposite sex, increased peer pressure, and the desire for more freedom
   • *Spiritual:* an overall sense "I want to get closer to God but I don't know how", or other questions about God's role in your own life

2. A teen experiences things so intensely because of all the changes taking place in his/her body: physical changes, emotional frustrations, social pressures, and spiritual concerns.

3. First, identify your worries, starting with the greatest one. After you realize what your greatest source of worry is right now, share it with God. As you are talking with God, take the time to listen to what He says to you in your mind and in your heart. He will give you a sense of peace about your concern. Next, talk to someone you can trust, preferably an adult.

4. God wants to mold you into the likeness of Jesus Christ—to become more like Him!

Applying the Truth

1. When a potter throws a pot, the clay must be of good quality (the clay represents your life). Each change to the piece brings it closer to what the artist (God) wants the pot to become. God never makes mistakes, and does not give up on a piece of clay! But the clay must cooperate and be pliable.

The purpose for the vessel has been determined before the potter begins his work on the piece. Once the artist believes the vessel needs strengthening or testing, it will go into the fire (difficult times for a Christian). Depending upon the purpose for the piece, the clay may have to experience the intense heat of the fire over and over again. But every time, if the clay does not crack under the pressure, it comes out stronger and more ready for use.

2. Sometimes bad things happen to Christians, just like non-Christians. Many times, you don't understand why things happen. There is no easy answer for this, but God has a unique way of causing good to come from bad. I know it is hard right now, but if you turn to God and share your true feelings, He will help you through this time.

3. Comparison and jealousy ruin relationships. They put a big wedge between you and the other person. They also affect your thoughts about yourself. Possibly worst of all, they can lead you into pride to think that you are better than others. If you have a problem with jealousy, talk to God about the way you feel and ask Him to help you overcome comparison and be grateful for all that He has done for you.

4. Answers may vary but the general theme for each illustration should include:

   • The Faithful Servant: Increase Your Personal Responsibilities. "He who is faithful in little will be faithful in much."

   • Samuel: Focus on What Really Matters. "Man looks on the outward, but God looks at the heart."

   • King David: Grow in Openness to God. "My God, my God, why have you forsaken me?"

   • Judas: Avoid Secrecy and Isolation. Judas "went out and it was night."

   • Joseph: Learn How to Forgive Those Who Hurt You. "You meant it for evil, but God meant it for good."

   • Peter: Stand-Alone Courage. "But Peter...raised his voice and said to them..."

Chapter 7 Review Answers

Defining the Terms

Distract: to divide the mind

Self-control: being able to restrain your words or behaviors that might hurt you or someone else

Boundary: an invisible line that separates you from everyone and everything else; like a fence with a gate that you control between you and the outside world

Goal: an achievement toward which you work; your personal aim, purpose, or end in doing or not doing something

Short-term goal: something that you make specific plans to accomplish within a relatively brief period of time

Long-term goal: something that you make specific plans to get done over a relatively long period of time

Recalling the Facts

1. Society values having a lot of money, fame, intelligence, and good looks.

   God values inner character qualities like self-control, love, kindness, obedience, respect, and wisdom.

2. 1) Make wise choices

   2) Stay mentally focused

   3) Gain self-control

   4) Develop appropriate boundaries

   5) Set realistic goals

   6) Become a lifelong learner

   7) Stay motivated

3. • Learn from others' experiences

   • Get input from mature adults you trust

   • Take time to think about your decisions

   • Pray for wisdom

Applying the Truth

1. • Homework: Turn off the TV and the music. Reward yourself when you reach small goals. Use a student calendar to stay organized. Study in the library instead of at home. Don't take any phone calls until after you have completed your work.

   • Chores around the house: Give yourself a time limit and pace yourself. Don't allow yourself to do anything 'fun' until your chores are done.

   • Finishing projects that you start: Set small goals for the project so it does not seem so overwhelming. Learn not to procrastinate. Work with another person. Be accountable to someone about your schedule.

   • Music lessons: Don't wait until you "feel" like practicing. Set the same time everyday to practice. Make it a part of your daily routine.

2. A boundary is an invisible barrier between you and the outside world. It helps to prevent you from hurting yourself physically or emotionally by making unwise choices that are outside your boundary. They stop you from hurting others feelings and they give you a way of protecting

yourself by being able confidently to say "No".

3. If you were to cheat on a math test, it would be a sin; but if you got an answer wrong on your math test because you forgot how to do the problem or did not understand, then it is a mistake but not a sin. A sin is a moral or spiritual transgression, contradictory to God's nature and His laws. A mistake, like missing a math problem, is not a sin (although you probably could have studied a little bit more!) Even though all sins are mistakes, all mistakes are not sins. If you sinned, repent and He will forgive you (*I John* 1:9). If you made a mistake that wasn't a sin, learn to accept your weaknesses; "live and learn".

4. Satan wants you to feel depressed, fearful and unmotivated to change. This keeps you away from God and others. Satan wants you to harden your heart, but God wants you to have a heart that is willing to change. When Satan tries to keep you away from God and others who might help you, God wants you to go to Him and others immediately and not to wait. God wants to help you learn from your mistakes and cause good to come from them.

Chapter 8 Review Answers

Defining the Terms

Social health: your ability to get along with different kinds of people

Friendship: a social connection in which people willingly share common interests or activities

Relationship: a tie with people by blood, marriage, work, or social role

Substitutions: replacing one person or thing with another

Artificial relationships: bonding with someone or something that doesn't really exist as an actual living person in real life

Communication: the act of expressing thoughts, feelings, information, or beliefs easily or effectively through speech, writing, media, or signs

Verbal communication: sharing a message through words or talking

Nonverbal communication: sharing a message without talking such as body language, hand motions, or facial expressions

A Wall: a barrier between people that hinders their communication

Infatuation: feeling temporary strong emotional attraction to a person of the opposite sex

Positive peer pressure: what you feel when others encourage you to do something that is good for you or others

Negative peer pressure: what you feel when others encourage you to do something that is harmful for you or others

Respect: esteem, admiration, acceptance, or courtesy; not intruding upon or interfering with another person's rights

Disrespect: lack of courtesy, rude, insulting, sarcastic, or sassy

Reputation: what people think of you

Revenge: wanting to get even with someone

Forgive: to release all of your desire to punish or get even with those who have hurt or offended you

Empathy: when you really feel for a person who is hurt because you've experienced the same hurt

Recalling the Facts

1. A computer program or game, a Hollywood actor or actress, a star athlete or the lives of those on a soap opera or sitcom can become artificial relationships for some teens. This is dangerous because it can promote isolation and a lack of accountability with others.

2. Jonathan and David (*I Samuel* 18:1-4) had a unique friendship because they shared deeply and openly with one another. They sacrificed for the good of the other person.

3. Communicating is expressing thoughts, feelings and information effectively. To do this, a person must learn to listen and understand the other person rather than just "talk" about his/her own opinions.

4. 1) Realize that first impressions can be misleading.

   2) Choose the right time and place.

   3) Know what your true feelings are—and stick to them.

   4) Avoid yelling, screaming, and name-calling.

   5) Be an active and sensitive listener.

   6) Be quick to apologize.

   7) Accept the person even if you reject the idea.

   8) Recognize walls in yourself and others.

   9) Use "I" statements instead of "You" statements.

   10) Describe the present situation only. Avoid statements that use the words "never" and "always".

   11) Accept the fact that some conflicts will take time to be resolved.

   12) Put yourself in the other person's place.

5. • Define what the purpose is for 'single dating'.

   • Know your level of maturity.

   • Know your parent's dating standards for you.

6. Develop good communication skills with your parents and mature, safe adults. When you invest in healthy friendships, you surround yourself with the positive influence of good friends. As a result, negative peer pressure won't affect you as much.

Applying the Truth

1. The words that you use to talk with others come from your heart and your mind. They include words you hear most of the time, from what kinds of music you listen to, and what kind of books you read. If you fill your mind and heart with nonsense words, nonsense words will be what you speak. But if you fill your mind and heart with godly words and thoughts, then these words will be communicated through your speech. Words can never be "taken back" and can hurt another person's feelings.

2. When a teen shows favoritism only to those who look good, wear designer clothes, have money, are intelligent, have athletic ability or have a cool car, they are showing partiality. God wants us to show unconditional respect to all people, Christian and non-Christian. God made each person in His image and for His own special purpose.

3. Gossips don't have many friends except for others who gossip. They can't keep their friends very long because they don't respect other people's private matters. Ask God to help you overcome the temptation to gossip. The next time you are around friends, practice saying something nice

about a person who is not with you and see what the response is in the group. Speaking positively about others is part of becoming more like Christ.

Chapter 9 Review Answers

Defining the Terms

Epidermis: the outer layer of skin

Dermis: the middle layer of skin

Subcutaneous layer: the deepest layer of skin

Acne: occurs when the pores of your skin become clogged with oil

Sebum: an oily substance that eventually clogs the pores of your skin

Whitehead: a type of acne that is created when oil becomes trapped inside a pore

Blackhead: a pore that's plugged with oil— but is exposed to the air

Pimple: a clogged pore that has become infected and filled with pus. Pimples are the most serious type of acne.

Dermatologist: a doctor who treats skin disorders

Follicle: The roots of your hair are secured in these small pockets.

Dandruff: a condition in which the outer layer of skin on the scalp flakes off

Head lice: insects that live in the hair and look very similar to dandruff

Keratin: a hard substance that gives nails their strength

Cuticle: surrounds the nail and is made of a nonliving skin. The cuticle protects the base of the nail from germs and bacteria.

Ingrown toenail: a nail that pushes into the skin on the side of your toe

Masticate: chew thoroughly

Periodontium: the name of the bone, tissue, and gum that support your teeth

Cavity: when bacteria combines with sugary foods and forms an acid

Plaque: a grainy, sticky coating that is constantly forming on your teeth

Tartar: a substance that hardens on your teeth

Gingivitis: a gum disease caused by a build-up of plaque and tartar on your teeth

Periodontal disease: more advanced gum disease

Malocclusion: when your upper and lower teeth don't line up properly

Orthodontics: braces can treat severe irregularities of the teeth

Halitosis: bad breath

Farsightedness: a condition where a person has difficulty seeing things that are close

Nearsightedness: a condition where a person has difficulty seeing things that are far away

Astigmatism: a condition in which a person's vision is distorted due to the irregular shape of the cornea or lens

Pink eye: a very contagious condition caused by a bacterial infection

Sty: when one of the small glands in your eyelid gets infected and swollen. It may look like a pimple.

Recalling the Facts

1. • Being clean and attractive will definitely enhance your looks, but try not to fall into the trap of always wanting to look good for other people.

   • Taking care of yourself makes you feel good about yourself.

   • Using good personal hygiene shows respect, not only to others, but also to yourself.

- Practicing good hygiene daily will boost your confidence in social situations and positively affect your relationship with others.

2. The worst time to be in the sun is between 10:00AM and 3:00PM. The sun is too intense for your skin and can cause a burn.

3. Do
   - Wash with a facial cleanser and warm water twice a day.
   - Dry your skin carefully with a clean towel. Don't scrub the area.
   - Use a mild cleanser suited to your skin type (to help control the excess oil).
   - Get plenty of rest.
   - Exercise regularly.
   - Eat fresh whole foods.
   - Drink more than eight glasses of purified water daily.
   - Wear oil-free make-up.
   - If your condition is serious, see a dermatologist (a doctor who treats skin disorders).
   - Understand that acne will eventually go away.

   Don't
   - Squeeze or pick at your acne. This can cause infection and scarring.
   - Use heavy creams or moisturizers on the affected areas.
   - Touch your face with your hands or fingers. This can place more oil and dirt on your face.
   - Let acne get you depressed or prevent you from having fun!

4. • First, try to stay calm. If you've ever changed your hairstyle—or got a 'fad' cut—then you know how it can affect your whole outlook on life. One good line to tell yourself after you get your hair cut is, "It'll always grow back!"

- Second, there are different types of hair. It's true that different hair types need different shampoos, conditioners, and cuts to maximize their style, but try not to stop there. Look at the shape of your head and face to help to determine what kind of style is right for you.
- Third, hairstyles change as often as clothing styles. Try not to pick the "in" cut if it's not the best for you. Find something that makes you feel good and confident about yourself and stick with it. Another good question to keep in mind about any new hairstyle is, "Is this style really practical for me?" If you have a hard time getting up in the morning, for example, try to stay away from a hairstyle that demands major styling time.

5. • Brush your teeth after each meal.
   - Brush your tongue.
   - Change your toothbrush.
   - Floss at least once a day.
   - Use fluoride.
   - Eat healthfully.
   - Visit your dentist twice a year.

6. In the center of the iris is the pupil.

7. The most common form of ear trouble is an ear infection. A viral or bacterial infection of the nose, throat, or Eustachian tubes can cause intense ear pain. Unlike a middle-ear infection, swimmer's ear occurs in the outer ear.

8. When sitting down, try always to have your seat and lower back pushed back up against the back of the chair. This will help to prevent undue stress on your lower back muscles and prevent lower back pain. Imagine a string with a helium balloon connected to the crown (the very highest part) of your head. Pretend the balloon is pulling straight upward. Your chin should go down and your neck come back into proper alignment with your shoulders. If you still have posture problems, imagine that same string and balloon on the front of your chest pulling your chest up and out.

9. • Take special note of how you feel when you bite your nails. Do you feel bored, nervous, or depressed? If so, the next time the urge hits, try telling yourself, "I need to find something else to do right away so that I don't feel bored, nervous, or depressed."
   - The next time the urge to bite them comes, try some of this self-talk: "I really don't have to bite them", or "Biting them isn't really worth it".
   - Try doing something else with your hands, for example, getting something to drink.
   - Make a decision to stop. Tell someone else who may hold you accountable and ask how you're doing.
   - Keep your nails trimmed and smooth so that you won't be tempted to bite them.
   - Give yourself a treat if you go one month without biting your nails. How about your favorite sundae or milk shake? How about a manicure?
   - Try a bitter-tasting polish (or liquid) so your nails will taste badly if you bite them.
   - If you still have problems, limit your biting to one nail.

Applying the Truth

1. God created your physical eyes to gather information. Your eyes, however, can receive both negative as well as positive input. It's important to protect

yourself from the damage caused by negative influences. Teenagers must be careful, with all the pressures of society, to protect their mind and heart. Images which teens allow into their minds affect their thought life as well as their attitudes.

2. Be quick to hear and slow to speak! It is more difficult to listen than it is to speak. When angry, you are more likely to speak first than be silent.

3. By keeping what comes into your eyes and ears as pure as possible; by using the G.I.G.O. principle to help you be more like Christ.

Chapter 10 Review Answers

Defining the Terms

Cirrhosis: a chronic disease of the liver that often results from a longstanding addiction to alcohol

Inhibitory effect: a result of alcohol that causes the blocking of the center of the brain that controls a person's degree of self-control and shyness

Alcoholism: an illness characterized by habitual, compulsive, long-term, and heavy drinking

Tolerance: a resistance in the body to something

Withdrawal: the physical disturbance that results when an individual does not consume a substance he/she is addicted to

MADD: Mothers Against Drunk Driving

Alcoholics Anonymous (AA): a support group specifically designed for alcoholics

Alateen: a group designed to help children of alcoholic parents

Al-Anon: a group designed to help the husbands, wives, and friends of alcoholics

Alexander Fleming: discovered the drug penicillin in London in 1928

Drugs: substances that alter the function of one or more body organs

Medicines: drugs that are meant to relieve pain, cure diseases, or prevent other illnesses

Drug abuse: a condition that occurs when a person uses an illegal drug or misuses a legal one

Prescription drugs: drugs that are sold only with a written order from a doctor

Nonprescription drugs: "over-the-counter" drugs that are medicines that can be sold without a doctor's written permission

FDA: The U.S. Food and Drug Administration tests drugs to make sure they are safe

Side effects: any reactions to a drug other than the intended effect

Caffeine: a stimulant

Stimulants: drugs that speed up the body's nervous system

Addiction: a physical or mental need for a drug or other substance

Depressants: drugs that tend to slow down your body's nervous system

Narcotics: a form of depressant that induces sleep or decreases feeling

Morphine and codeine: highly addictive narcotics that are prescribed as painkillers

Heroin: an illegal drug that is a depressant and is extremely dangerous

PCP or angel dust (phencyclidine): an extremely dangerous hallucinogen

LSD (lysergic acid diethylamide): an extremely dangerous hallucinogen

Hallucinogen: a group of drugs that cause the brain to form unreal images

Inhalants: substances whose fumes are breathed in to give the user a high-like feeling; can cause permanent brain damage

Denial: refusing to acknowledge the existence of a problem

Nicotine: a colorless, oily, water-soluable, highly toxic and addictive, liquid alkaloid obtained from tobacco

Tar: a thick, dark, sticky liquid that is formed when tobacco burns

Carbon monoxide: a poisonous gas that is produced by car engines and burning tobacco

Emphysema: an irreversible lung disease that is primarily caused by smoking

Second-hand smoke (passive smoke): the smoke you breathe that comes from another person's smoking

Mainstream smoke: the smoke that is inhaled and then exhaled by the smoker

Sidestream smoke: the smoke that comes out of the end of a lit cigarette

Environmental smoke: the smoke that stays in the air where smokers have been smoking

Recalling the Facts

1. Show responsibility, gain more freedom; show more responsibility, gain more freedom. Freedom is something that a teenager earns, not demands.

2. • Increased freedom gives teens more time and exposure to learn about substances. Increased curiosity from asking questions such as, "What would it be like?"

   • More freedom gives teens a greater opportunity to discover and express their own individuality.

3. • Slurred speech

- Inability to walk straight
- Forgetfulness
- Acting obnoxious
- Endangering themselves or others
- Assaulting someone
- Embarrassing themselves

4. Advertiser's promote the pleasures and 'cool' image associated with the use of tobacco, alcohol, and other products that are dangerous to your health. You don't see a commercial of a person experiencing a hangover from drinking too much.

5. Coffee, tea and many soda pops are high in caffeine that is a stimulant. Caffeine increases the body's nervous system which can cause withdrawal symptoms. People who drink a lot of pop, tea, and coffee and then go without it, may experience headaches, weakness and a general sense of mental distraction from the body's strong craving. The more you drink a caffeinated beverage, the greater your body's demand for it will be.

6. • Causes irregular heartbeat
- Increases hunger
- Slows down the body's rate of development
- Lowers body temperature
- Impairs perception and response time
- Damages the immune system
- Hurts the reproductive system
- Injures brain cells
- Causes the user to view reality in a distorted way

7. Just one try of a drug can start a lifetime of addiction. Drugs today are more potent and dangerous than years ago. One try can end in death.

8. Possible answers may be:
- Curiosity

- Look cool
- Peer pressure
- Want to feel a "buzz"
- Want to rebel against their parent's rules
- Think they will quit when they get older
- Feel indestructible ("I'll never get cancer. Other people smoke, and they're still living.")

Applying the Truth

1. To make it through today's culture you must have your own personal convictions (strong beliefs). You cannot rely only upon what your parents believe. You must have your own personal relationship with God and begin to make your own decisions based on the Scriptures about the issues that confront you.

2. • Avoid an argument with your parents (*Proverbs* 17:14);
- Have lots of friends (*Proverbs* 18:24);
- Earn money for a bike or a car (*Proverbs* 10:4);
- Choose the best boyfriend (*Proverbs* 22:24); and,
- Choose the best girlfriend and wife (*Proverbs* 19:14; 31:10-31).

3. • Since God is love (*I John* 4:16), He wants you to experience His love so that you can show it to others.
- Since one of the fruit of the Spirit is joy (*Galatians* 5:22) and, as David wrote to God, "In Your presence is fullness of joy" (*Psalm* 16:11), He wants you to feel His joy inside of your heart so that you can share it.
- Since one of the fruit of the Spirit is peace (*Galatians* 5:22), Paul recommends when you are full of anxiety, "Let your requests be made known to God" (*Philippians*

4:6), so that you can know, "... the peace of God that surpasses all understanding [which] will guard your hearts and minds through Christ Jesus" (*Philippians* 4:7).
- Since Jesus has all supernatural power at His disposal (*Matthew* 28:17), He wants you to encounter some of His power so that you can help a hurting and dying world.

Chapter 11 Review Answers

Defining the Terms

Comprehension: understanding and remembering what you've read

Intellectual: mental; having to do with your mind

Regress: to go backward

Humility: realizing your own limitations

Hypocrites: "two-faced", giving the impression that you have certain beliefs, or feelings that you really don't have

Countenance: the expression of your face

Recalling the Facts

1. • Martin Luther, church reformer
- John Calvin, church reformer
- John Wycliffe, church reformer, Bible translator
- Charles Finney, evangelist
- John Wesley, founder of Methodism

2. • The next time you watch a movie, look at the credits and see what book the movie was taken from. Many—if not most—movies come from already-published books. Read the book upon which your favorite movie was based. Compare the book with the movie.

- Tell yourself that you're going to spend just as much time reading as you do watching TV or movies.
- Try not using any electronic entertainment for a day, a week, or more. See if you get better grades, develop more friendships, have fun learning something new, or get more good books read.
- Find a friend who likes to read the same kind of books that you do.
- Use a Bible translation that you really understand and like.
- Help to put together a home environment that is favorable to reading.

3. Questions are good as long as they come from a heart that is simply seeking the truth. An attitude of pride, trying to be obnoxious, or trying to make someone be embarrassed or "look bad" are ways that questioning can be wrong. Check your motives and the timing of when to ask what question.

4. •Looking at them when they're talking to you;
- Acknowledging what they've said to you by repeating it back to them, or saying "Yes, Mom";
- Asking them to reconsider by giving them a good reason if you are struggling with what they've just asked you to do;
- Saying, "Please" more often; and
- Showing a grateful spirit toward all that they have done for you by saying "Thank you" more often.

5. One of the ways that you can show respect for your parents is in allowing them to "save face". As you mature, you're going to make some mistakes and so are your parents. Your parents have a lot of pressure on

them to "be right" and "do right" most of the time. Because of this pressure, they usually won't appreciate it if you expose their mistakes in a direct or disrespectful way; some won't like it at all. But, as you get older, you're going to see legitimate problems in your parents. The fact is that everybody has weaknesses because we're all fallen and broken human beings in need of God.

Applying the Truth

1. Answers will vary.
2. • What was it like when you were a teen?
- What jobs did you have when you were a teen?
- Do you have any idea(s) of what kind of job(s) I could get?
- I know that I'll be making my own decision, but what kind of career do you think that I might be good at?
- What kind of relationship did you have with your Dad or Mom? Did you ever get into any struggles or arguments with them? If so, about what? How did you resolve them?
- If you were to relive your teen years, what would you do the same? What would you do differently?
- Did you ever struggle with your faith in God?

Chapter 12 Review Answers

Defining the Terms

Prayer: talking to God and listening to hear what God would say to you

Fear: concern or anxiety about something real or imagined

Influence: the power of a person or thing to persuade or take advantage of you

Destiny: the purpose for which God has created you

Recalling the Facts

1. What your parents, teachers, and pastors have taught you about God is likely to be the same way that you think about Him. If your parents are easy to talk to and very understanding, you'll probably see God in that way, too. But, if your parents are distant or too busy for you, you might begin to think that God is the same way—even though He isn't.

2. • To help you to love God more (develop a closer relationship with Him).
- To show you how to love people more (like Jesus loves them).

3. Keeping your prayer "hot-line" open to God all day. Talking to God, even briefly, throughout your day. Thanking Him as well as asking Him for guidance.

4. Many of them only take one step at a time. This is the way the characters in the Bible lived, too. Why doesn't God show you a complete picture of your life all at once? It's because He wants you to learn to live by faith; to trust Him to put together each piece of your Life Puzzle in His own time and in His own way. If you're not sure what your next step is in fulfilling your special purpose, then start asking Him, and He'll begin to let you know. God's more anxious for you to discover His unique plan for you than you are to discover it!

Applying the Truth

1. One of the subtle ways that the enemy will use to try to get you to compromise your standards is to get you involved

with friends who have a negative influence upon you.

2. Satan loves to get you to sin. He knows that if he can make you feel so bad about yourself, you won't tell anyone and you will stay away from your loving Father. He will lie to you about yourself. He wants you to believe terrible things about how others and God feel about you. Don't believe him! You can expect opposition from Satan if you really want to make things right. He will lie to you about how bad you are and how disappointed God and others are in you. Don't listen to him! *James* 4:7. Humble yourself and go directly to God and those whom you have offended. As a result, you will grow in your spiritual maturity and feel like a brand new person!

3. All of these aspects that teens don't like about being a Christian make following Jesus challenging and sometimes difficult. Some teens decide that becoming a Christian is too hard and choose not to believe.

Others may pretend to love and serve God on the outside while inside they really don't want to pay the price to serve God. Consequently, they know how to "act" spiritual, yet lack a true relationship with Him. If you don't want to be a Christian "pretender", then ask the Lord to help you to know and love Him so much that you become willing to accept the things that you don't like about Christianity. In doing this, you'll be counting the cost of being a true follower of Jesus.

I think that the Lord is disappointed and sad when a person fakes having a relationship with Him. He desires a real relationship with each person and knows that really knowing Him is the way to true happiness.

4. • Through the Bible
   • In my heart
   • Through other people (parents)
   • Through the Holy Spirit
   • Through worship
   • In my conscience
   • In my dreams
   • Through my experiences